Zeineb Teyeb
Mariem Essouri
Naziha Khammassi

Therapeutic education in Sjögren's syndrome

Zeineb Teyeb
Mariem Essouri
Naziha Khammassi

Therapeutic education in Sjögren's syndrome

How do I manage my dry syndrome?

ScienciaScripts

Imprint

Any brand names and product names mentioned in this book are subject to trademark, brand or patent protection and are trademarks or registered trademarks of their respective holders. The use of brand names, product names, common names, trade names, product descriptions etc. even without a particular marking in this work is in no way to be construed to mean that such names may be regarded as unrestricted in respect of trademark and brand protection legislation and could thus be used by anyone.

Cover image: www.ingimage.com

This book is a translation from the original published under ISBN 978-620-6-72504-6.

Publisher:
Sciencia Scripts
is a trademark of
Dodo Books Indian Ocean Ltd. and OmniScriptum S.R.L publishing group

120 High Road, East Finchley, London, N2 9ED, United Kingdom
Str. Armeneasca 28/1, office 1, Chisinau MD-2012, Republic of Moldova, Europe
Printed at: see last page
ISBN: 978-620-3-35828-5

Contents

1 INTRODUCTION

Sjogren's syndrome (SS) or Gougerot-Sjogren's syndrome is a systemic autoimmune disease characterised by lymphoid infiltration of the salivary and lacrimal glands associated with the production of various autoantibodies [1].

The clinical picture is dominated by dry mouth or xerostomia and dry eyes or xerophthalmia. The dry syndrome, fatigue and polyarthralgias constitute a triad strongly suggestive of Sjogren's syndrome. In addition to the clinical dry syndrome, which may involve all the exocrine glands, systemic manifestations are often present: articular (75%), respiratory (75%), muscular (33%), cutaneous (30%), neurological (25 to 30%) and renal (20%). Hematological involvement is less frequent, apart from lymphopenia. Digestive manifestations, apart from dysphagia, are rare and not very specific [1].

Sjogren's syndrome may be primary or associated with another autoimmune disease such as systemic lupus erythematosus, rheumatoid arthritis, scleroderma, inflammatory myopathies or dysthyroTdies...

Given the clinical and paraclinical complexity of Sjogren's syndrome, several diagnostic criteria have been developed. The most recently published criteria are those proposed by the Sjogren International Collaborative Clinical Alliance (SICCA) expert group in 2012, but which are not yet valid [2]. Other criteria were developed in 2015 by the American College of Rheumatology (ACR) and the European League Against Rheumatism (EULAR) but have not yet been published. To date, most disease experts have agreed to use the 2002 American European Consensus Group (AECG) criteria [3]. In addition to the subjective signs of dry syndrome, these require objective criteria of immunological involvement, including lymphoid infiltration greater than or equal to Chisholm stage 3 on biopsy of the accessory salivary glands and/or the presence of anti-SSA or anti-SSB autoantibodies. Sjogren's syndrome is considered to exist when 4 criteria are present, including at least one criterion of immunological involvement (Appendix I).

The clinical manifestations of SS are numerous and vary in severity, but the dry syndrome remains the patient's main functional complaint. Apart from the functional gene, xerostomy is responsible for oral and dental complications (gingivitis, stomatitis, tooth decay, edentation that is difficult to remove, papillary atrophy, candidal infection, bacterial superinfection of the salivary glands, etc.).

Lifestyle measures aimed at avoiding aggravation of the dry syndrome are systematically recommended, such as avoiding smoking, dry conditions and certain medications (Appendix II). Local therapies, mainly artificial saliva or spray preparations, have been proposed but have proved disappointing. General therapeutics such as bromhexine and anetholtrithione have been known for years, but their efficacy is inconsistent and limited. Other molecules, such as pilocarpine and cevimeline, are currently recommended but are associated with essentially anticholinergic side-effects that are often perceived as annoying by patients (sweating, palpitations, flu syndrome, rhinitis, headache, pollakiuria, abdominal pain).

The availability of different molecules in our country makes the management of dry syndrome difficult. In Tunisia, only bromhexine is available on the market. Anetholtrithone and pilocarpine are available in Europe and America. Cevimeline is available in Japan and America. Preparations and sprays are not available either. Moreover, the cost of these products is high.

Some patients use olive oil (HO) as a topical treatment for gingivitis or stomatitis, in line with our traditions and customs. The virtues of HO have been known for decades. Countries with a Mediterranean diet have fewer cardiovascular events and a longer life expectancy, thanks in large part to a diet rich in olive oil. The quality of Tunisian olive oil is recognised by olive growing experts and is among the best in the world [4]. Local application of olive oil has emollient properties [5]. Several recent studies have looked at the anti-inflammatory and antioxidant activity of HO applied generically. In the same context of ancestral phytotherapy, some patients with SS have tried HO to relieve their dry mouth. No Tunisian or international study has evaluated the benefit of using HO on xerostomia as a local treatment, whatever the etiology. This prompted us to study the effect of olive oil as a mouthwash on xerostomia in patients with **Sjogren**'s syndrome (the **HOSS** study).

The aim of our study in patients with SS was to compare the percentages of improvement in xerostomia with HO mouthwash combined with usual treatment compared with usual treatment alone based on the hypothesis of

Significant improvement in xerostomia in at least 40% of patients treated with a combination of mouthwashes with HO and the usual treatment compared with the usual treatment alone.

A counter-hypothesis stating that an improvement in xerostomia of less than 40% would be clinically uninteresting is inaccurate, because even an improvement of more than the indicated rate is still clinically interesting, given the availability and safety of the product.

I. Type of study :

This is a prospective, randomised, crossover, single-blind, bi-centric study conducted over 6 months (January 2015 to June 2015).

In order to ensure group comparability, simple randomisation was performed. A pre-established randomisation list was drawn up (Appendix III). Patients randomised to "A" received HO in 1ere period and their usual treatment alone in 2eme period. The periods were reversed in the case of randomisation "B".

II. Study population :

The files of patients with SS followed at the CHU Mongi Slim La Marsa and at the regional hospital of Ben Arous were studied. Patients meeting the criteria of the AECG 2002 were contacted to confirm the possibility of inclusion.

1. Inclusion criteria :

^ Prior agreement to participate in the therapeutic trial.

^ Adult patients with primary or associated SS diagnosed according to the criteria of the AECG 2002 group **AND** with a xerostomy assessed by the Eular Sjogren's Syndrome Patient Reported Index (ESSPRI) score with a dryness score greater than or equal to 5 and who have given their written informed consent to participate in the study presented by the investigator.

^ SS evolving for 6 months or more.

2. Non-inclusion criteria :

Age under 20
Refusal to take part in the study
Inability to give informed consent
Medical file not found
Patient lost to follow-up or unreachable
Patients with active neoplasia
SS not meeting CETA 2002 criteria
Patient without xerostomy gene
Xerostomy assessed by an ESSPRI score of less than 5
Known allergy to HO
SS evolving for less than 6 months
Exclusion criteria from the AECG 2002 diagnostic criteria (history of cervical irradiation, infection with hepatitis C virus or human immunodeficiency virus, pre-existing lymphoma, sarcoidosis, graft versus host disease, use of anticholinergic drugs).

3. Exclusion criteria :

s Intolerance to HO

s Occurrence of an intercurrent condition affecting the application of HO or affecting the evaluation of the effect of HO.

s Occurrence of neoplasia or a condition covered by the AECG 2002 exclusion criteria.

III. Informed consent:

Participants were given written informed consent in both English and Arabic. The investigating physician clearly explained the points of the consent without influencing the patient. The participant was free to give or withhold consent. The patient was included as soon as written consent was signed (Appendix IV and V).

IV. Ethics Committee :

The therapeutic trial was approved by the ethics committees of the Mongi Slim Hospital and the Ben Arous Regional Hospital after presentation of the study protocol (Appendices VI and VII).

V. Conflict of interest :

All the investigators have no conflicts of interest.

VI. Treatment : Olive oil

1. International designations :

The olive tree or Olea Europea L. (Figure 1), a typical Mediterranean tree, is characterised by its fruit, the olive.

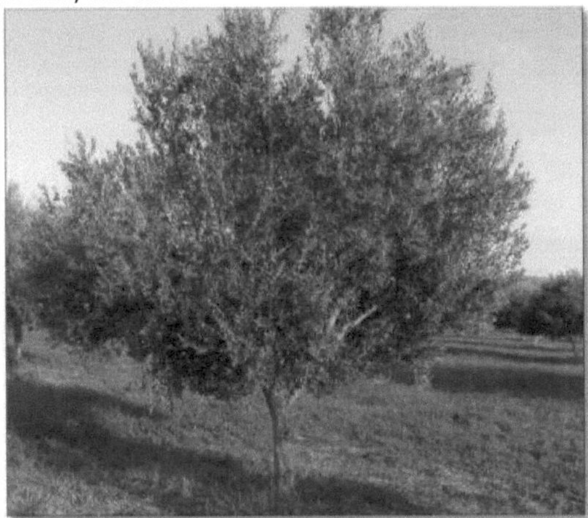

Figure 1: Olive tree in the Ben Arous region.

The vernacular names of the olive tree, the olive and olive oil are summarised in Table I [5,6].

Table I: Vernacular names for the olive tree, the olive and olive oil.

	olive tree	Olive	olive oil
Arabic	Chajaret azzeitoun	zeitouna	Zayt ezzeitoune
French	Olive	olive	Olive oil
English	Olivetree	olive	Olive oil
Turkish	Zeytin	zeytin	Zeytinyagi
German	Olbauman	Olive	Olivenol
Italian	Ulivo	olivo	Olio d'oliva
Spanish	Olivo	aceituna	Aceita de oliva
Portuguese	Oliveira	azeitona	Azeite

2. Botany :

The cultivated olive tree is a hardy tree, 5 to 10 metres high, with a sinuous trunk whose crevices have lanceolate leaves and fruits of varying shape and oil content depending on the species (Figure 2) [7].

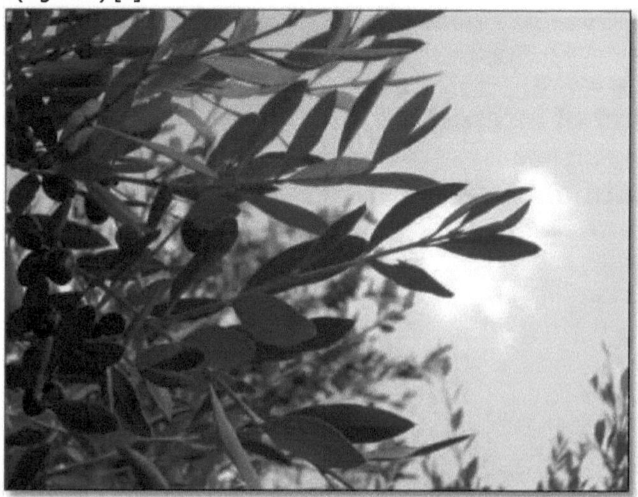

Figure 2: Leaves and fruit of the olive tree.

The botanical status of the species is detailed in Table II.

Table II: Botanical situation of the species Olea europea L.

Regne	Plantae
Branch	Magnoliophyta
Sub-branch	Magnoliophytina
Class	Magnoliopsida
Subclass	Dialypetals
Order	Lamiales
Family	Oleacecae
Type	Olea
Species	Olea europea L.
Sub-species	O. europea subsp. Europea var. sylvestris
	O. europea subsp. Europea var. Europea

The olive tree is exceptionally long-lived. A hundred-year-old olive tree is a tree in full production. The olive, the fruit of the olive tree, is a smooth-skinned drupe with a fleshy shell enclosing a very hard stone containing a seed (Figure 3).

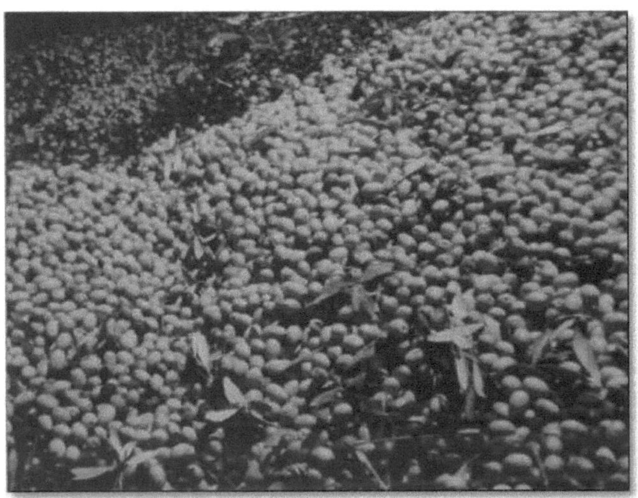
Figure 3: Freshly picked olives.

Olive oil is obtained by crushing the fruit in a special oil mill. The composition of the oil varies according to the area, local agronomic practices, variety and stage of ripeness at harvest. It should be kept cool and protected from light [5,6,8].

3. Main characteristics of the olive oil chosen :

The HO chosen is a Tunisian oil of international renown, exhibited at several international olive-growing shows. The harvest region is the Sahel, but the sub-species of olive trees used could not be specified because the producer contacted on several occasions refused to reply.

An analysis of the composition, the quality and a sensory study of the selected HO was carried out at the Office National de l'Huile according to the analysis methods adopted by the International Olive Oil Council (IOOC) (Annex VIII).

3.1. Composition:

The fatty acid composition by gas chromatography of the selected olive oil is detailed in Table III.

Table III: Chemical composition of the selected olive oil.

Fatty Acid	COI T20 Doc24*, Doc17t
Oleic acid	58.39
Linoleic acid	17.90
Palmitic acid	17.52
Stearic acid	2.37
Palmitoleic acid	2.36
Linolenic acid	0.69
Arachidic acid	0.42
Gadoleic acid	0.20
Hepthadecanoic acid	0.05
Hepthadecenoic acid	0.09

*Preparation of methyl esters of fatty acids

+ Determination of trans isomer fatty acids by capillary column gas chromatography analysis

3.2. Quality :

The free acidity content expressed as oleic acid is 0.73% (ISO 660). The peroxide value is 17 Meg/Kg.

3.3. Sensory analysis :

The sensory analysis concluded that it was virgin olive oil. There was a one-month delay between the sample being sent to the national oil office and its chemical characteristics being studied.

4. Undesirable effects :

Chronic inhalation of olive oil can lead to long-term oily pneumonitis [9]. Patients were not exposed to this undesirable effect as the product is applied locally to the mouth and not inhaled.

5. Toxicity :

No toxicity has been reported. However, it is important to point out that olive oil from non-organic production close to oil-producing areas or industrially refined may contain high levels of highly carcinogenic polycyclic aromatic hydrocarbons [10,11].

6. Contraindications:

None apart from a known allergy to olive oil [6].

7. How to use :

A sample of HO delivered in a 120 ml glass bottle was given to the participant. The patient used the equivalent of one teaspoon of HO as a mouthwash for at least 5 minutes, twice a day, in the morning after breakfast and in the evening before bedtime after usual oral hygiene, for 3 weeks. Using the amount taken from the teaspoon and the tip of his finger, he also applied the HO to his lips with the same frequency.

During the 3 weeks of usual treatment alone, no therapeutic changes were made.

The 3-week period was chosen because the duration of the various studies of local treatments for xerostomia varied between 7 and 28 days. In addition, a pre-study involving 10 patients showed that 3 weeks was sufficient to observe a benefit from topical application of HO.

VII. Assessment tools

In this study, we used specific tools (sicca Baseline questionnaire, Eular Sjogren's Syndrome Patient Reported Index and Xerostomia inventory) and non-specific tools (Visual Analogue Scale and oral cavity examination). All patients were assessed by the same examiner.

1. Specific tools :

1.1. Sicca baseline questionnary :

The questionnaire consisted of 70 multiple response questions. It was divided into 7 sections (demographics, ethnicity, smoking status, overall physical and emotional evaluation, gynaeco-obstetric antecedents, oral symptoms and ocular symptoms). This questionnaire is valid for therapeutic trials [12].

The questions were asked in dialectical Arabic or in French for French-speaking patients

(Appendices IX and X). The Arabic version was not previously validated and was translated for the purposes of the study.

1.2. Eular Sjogren's Syndrome Patient Reported Index (ESSPRI) :

It is a valid tool for clinical trials assessing dryness, fatigue and pain in patients with Sjogren's syndrome [13].

The patient answered the following question: "How would you rate the intensity of your (symptom) over the last 2 weeks? The patient was asked to quantify his gene by a number from 0 to 10. Zero corresponded to the absence of the symptom and 10 to the maximum of the gene. The sum of the 3 numbers attributed to each symptom constituted the total ESSPRI score. The most severe score possible is 30.

The questions were asked in dialectical Arabic or in French for French-speaking patients (Appendices XI and XII). The Arabic version was not previously validated and was translated for the purposes of the study.

1.3. Xerostomia Inventory (XI) :

This is a valid score for assessing dry mouth, consisting of 11 items:

- I drink water to swallow food
- My mouth feels dry when I eat
- I wake up at night to drink water
- My mouth feels dry
- I find it hard to eat certain foods
- I suck sweets or eat chewing gum to relieve my dry mouth
- I have difficulty swallowing certain foods
- The skin on my face is dry
- I have dry eyes
- My lips are dry
- I have a dry nose

The intensity of these symptoms was rated: Never (1 point), Hardly ever (2 points), Occasionally (3 points), Often (4 points) and Frequently (5 points).

The sum of the item ratings is the XI score. The minimum score is 11. The maximum possible score is 55 [14].

These questions were asked in dialectical Arabic or in French for French-speaking patients (Appendices XIII and XIV). The Arabic version was not previously validated and was translated for the purposes of the study.

Four of the 11 questions in the Xerostomia Inventory are directly related to xerostomia: I feel a dry mouth when I eat, I wake up at night to drink water, I feel a dry mouth and My lips are dry.

In order to better target oral dryness, we have considered these items as a mini-XI.

2. Non-specific tools :

2.1. Visual Analogue Scale (VAS) :

This scale is used to assess the global activity of the pathology lost by the patient. This scale is validated for therapeutic trials [15]. A visual scale from 0 to 10 was presented to the patient to answer the question "How would you rate the overall activity of your disease over the last 2 weeks? Zero corresponds to no activity and 10 to the maximum disease activity imagined by the patient.

2.2. Examination of the oral cavity :

A pre-established table was allocated to each patient included. It was marked with a "+" if the description was present and with a "-" if it was not (Appendix XV).

The oral cavity examination was carried out by the same investigator (internist in training).

It specified the following characteristics:

- Dry, sticky mucous membrane
- Dental caries
- Problems with wearing a prosthesis
- Generalized erythema of the oral mucosa
- Erythema as a geographical map of the oral mucosa
- Papillary atrophy
- Fissure of the dorsal surface of the tongue
- Erythema of the tongue
- Cheilitis at the corners of the mouth
- Chronic candidiasis
- Parotid tumour

3. An identification sheet :

Each patient included in the study had a unique identification form summarising all epidemiological data, glandular manifestations, extra-glandular manifestations, accessory salivary gland biopsy, immunological work-up, AECG 2002 and SICCA 2012 diagnostic criteria and treatment received (Appendix XVI).

VIII.   Schema of the study :

Each patient received 3 medical visits and at least one telephone call. The telephone call confirmed that the patient could be included after a review of the medical records. The 3 visits were carried out at inclusion, 3 weeks and 6 weeks.

Written informed consent was signed by the patient at the 1ere visit. Randomisation was carried out upon confirmation of inclusion. Data were collected using the above-mentioned tools.

The Xerostomia Inventory, ESSPRI, EVA and oral cavity examination were repeated at 2eme and 3eme contacts.

Figure 4 shows the experimental design of the HOSS study.

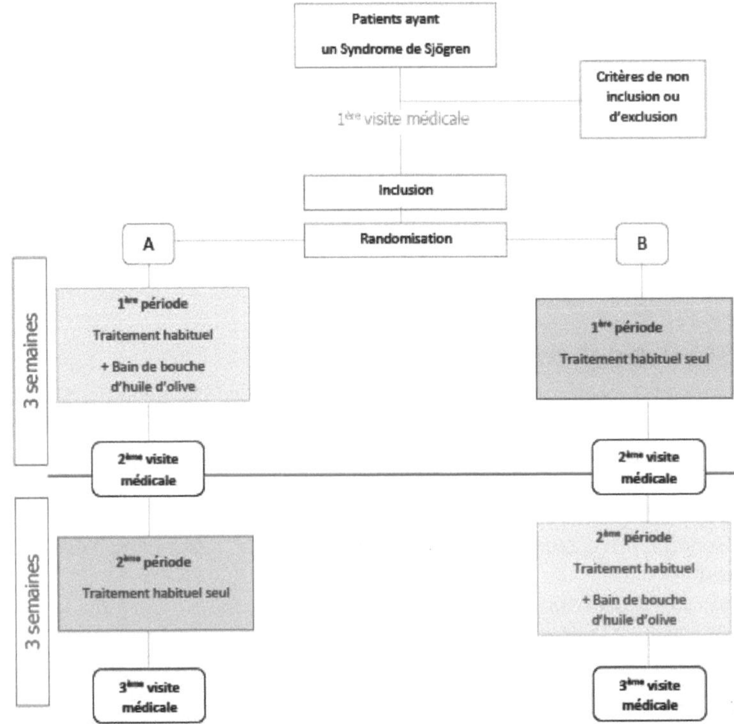

Figure 4: Diagram of the study.

IX. Judging criteria :

1. Primary endpoint :

These were considered significant:

^ Improvement in oral dryness detected by the 1^{iere} ESSPRI question on oral dryness > 20%.

and / or

J Decrease in Xerostomia Inventory score of at least 3 points

2. Secondary assessment criteria :

J Improvement in oral cavity examination (reduction or disappearance of an examination anomaly)

J EVA reduced by 25mm

X. Calculation of the number of subjects required:

In the absence of therapeutic modification, dry mouth was stable outside the first few months. Patients whose symptoms had been evolving for less than 6 months were not included. This allows us to say that for the patients included, the probability of spontaneous improvement without any therapeutic intervention tends towards zero.

The following formula is used to calculate the number of patients required for a crossover trial.

$$N' = \frac{N}{2}(1 - \varphi')$$

N': number of subjects in the event of cross-over

N : number of subjects required with 2 groups of patients

φ' : Correlation coefficient between the responses of the same subject to the 2 treatments

Since spontaneous recovery is rare or impossible, the difference in the endpoint between the two groups is significant. For a risk B at 5% and a <5%, the necessary number of patients is 12.

XI. Statistical study :

Comparisons of 2 means on independent series were carried out using the Student's t-test for independent series, and in the case of small numbers by the non-parametric Mann-Whitney test. Comparisons of 2 means on paired series were performed using the Student's t-test for paired series, and in the case of numbers < 30 by the non-parametric Wilcoxon test for paired series.

Comparisons of percentages on independent series were made using Pearson's chi-square test.

Comparisons of 2 percentages on matched series were carried out using the Mac Nemar test, and in the event of non-validity of this test, using the properties of the binomial distribution.

In all statistical tests, the significance level was set at 0.05.

The statistical analysis software used is Excel 2013 and SPSS version 22.

XII. Bibliographic research :

The bibliographic search was carried out on Pubmed, Sciendirect and Clinicalkey using the key words: Sjogren's syndrome, Gougerot-Sjogren's syndrome, xerostomy, Sjogren's syndrome, xerostomia, xerostomy treatment, olive oil, olea europea.

A/ Descriptive study

I. Conduct of the HOSS study :

Thirty-two patients were included over a total period of 6 months (January 2015 to June 2015). The last inclusion was on 4 May 2015. The last visit was on 16 June 2015. No inclusion errors were noted. No retraction after signed agreement to participate was requested. One patient with Sjogren's syndrome associated with anti-synthetase syndrome was excluded due to an episode of infectious pneumonitis causing the patient to discontinue HO of her own accord. One patient was lost to follow-up on the third contact.

1. Randomisation :

Patients were randomised equally between 1ere and 2eme periods, with 16 patients in each period.

2. Schema of the study :

Figure 5 summarises the conduct of the therapeutic trial.

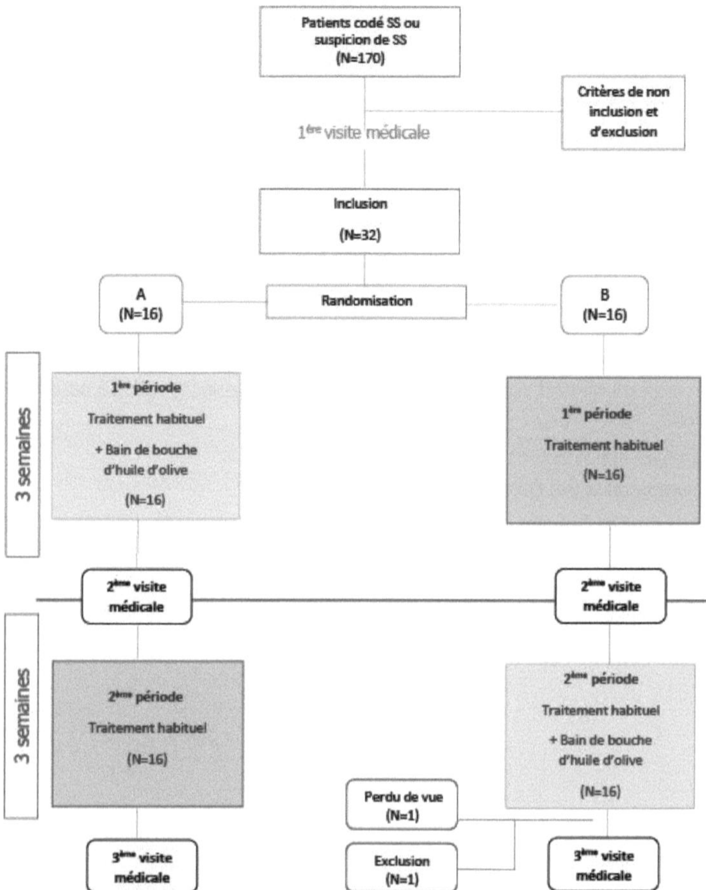

Figure 5: HOSS study process.

3. Month of olive oil application:

The distribution of patients according to the month of application of olive oil is shown below.

in Figure 6.

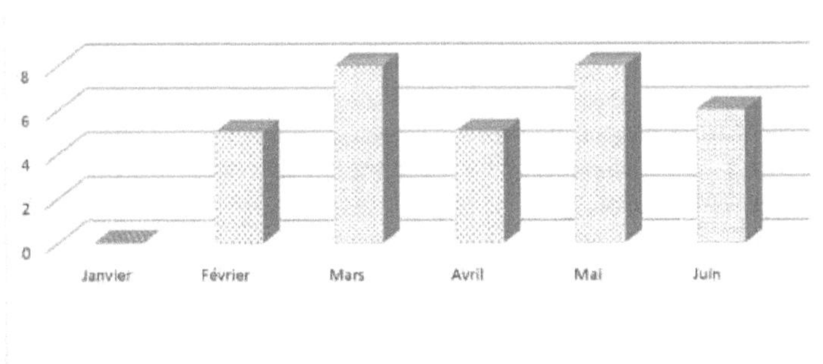

Figure 6 : Distribution of patients by month of olive oil application.

4. Cost of the study :

Seven litres of HO were purchased from supermarkets at a total cost of 80 Tunisian dinars.

Analysis of the physico-chemical characteristics of the selected HO cost 174 Tunisian dinars and 340 millimes (Annex XVII).

The glass bottles cost 20 Tunisian dinars.

This represents a total self-financing cost of 274 Tunisian dinars and 340 millimes.

11. Epidemiology :

1. Age :

The mean age was 51.6 ± 13.38 years, with extremes ranging from 28 to 73 years.

2. Genre :

The gender ratio was 0.1. There were 3 men and 29 women (Figure 7).

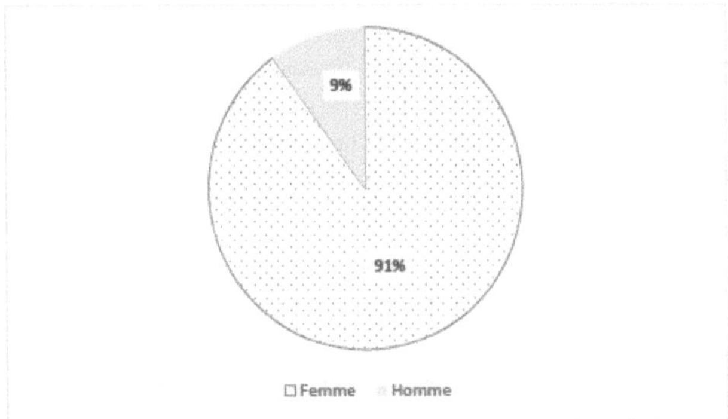

□ Female   Male

Figure 7: Breakdown of patients by gender.

3. Family history of autoimmune diseases:

Two patients had a family history of autoimmune disease. One patient had a history of

15

autoimmune peripheral hypothyroidism in the father. The other patient had several autoimmune diseases in the offspring: vitiligo, Biermer's anemia, alopecia and autoimmune peripheral hypothyroidism.

4. Personal history:

Four patients had no antecedents. Eight patients were being treated for a single medical condition other than SS. Twenty-four patients had 2 or more medical antecedents.

The patients' personal antecedents are summarised in Table IV.

Table IV: Personal history.

Antecedents	Number of patients	Percentage
Autoimmune pathology	13	40
Arterial hypertension	9	28
Rheumatological conditions	8	25
Ear, nose and throat pathology	6	18
Psychiatric condition	6	18
Allergies	6	18
Diabetes	5	15
Neoplasia	1	3
Cardiovascular event	1	1
Other	14	43

Psychiatric antecedents were distributed as follows: anxiety syndromes (n=2) and depressive syndromes (n=4).

Rheumatological antecedents were as follows: gonarthrosis (n=2), lumbosciatica (n=2), osteoporosis (n=2), hyper laxity of the patellar tendon in one patient and one case of cervicobrachial neuralgia.

Otorhinolaryngological antecedents were as follows: infectious pathologies (n=2), thyroid pathologies (n=2), a tonsillectomy and an acoustic neuroma.

The autoimmune pathologies collected are described in Figure 8.

Two patients had more than one autoimmune disease. One patient had primary biliary cirrhosis and autoimmune hemolytic anemia. The other patient had systemic scleroderma, Biermer's anemia and autoimmune peripheral hypothyroidism.

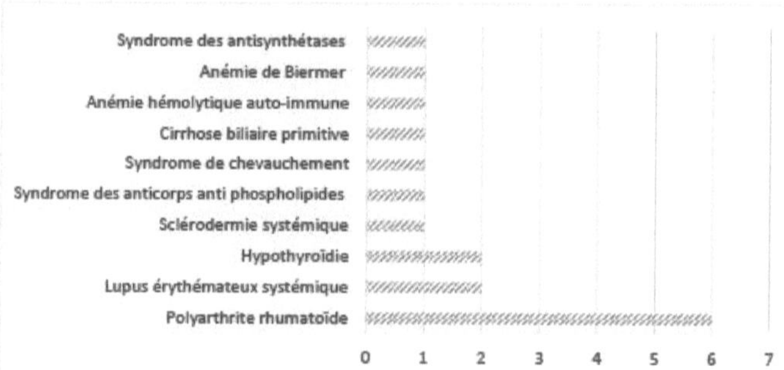

Antisynth^tase syndrome
Biermer's Апётне

Апётпе autoimmune h^molytic disease
Primary biliary cirrhosis
Overlap syndrome
Anti-phospholipid antibody syndrome
Systëmic sc^roderma
Hypothyroi'die
Systëmic lupus ërythëmateux
Rheumatoid arthritis
01234567

Figure 8: Associated autoimmune diseases.

5. Current treatment other than Sjogren :

The list of treatments received by patients is detailed in table V.

Table V: Treatments for patients other than Sjogren's syndrome.

Medicines	Number of patients
Metformin	4
Renin angiotensin system inhibitor	5
Calcium inhibitor	3
Non-steroidal anti-inflammatory drugs	3
Proton pump inhibitors	3
Hydroxychloroquine	3
Fibrates /statins	2 / 1
Serotonin reuptake inhibitors / psychotropic drugs	1 / 2
Hypoglycemic sulphonamides	1
Antihistamines	1
Chlorothiazide	1

111. Characteristics of Sjogren's syndrome :

112. Primitive or associated :

The distribution of patients according to the primary or associated nature of the SS diagnosis according to the criteria of the 2002 AECG group is shown in Figure 9.

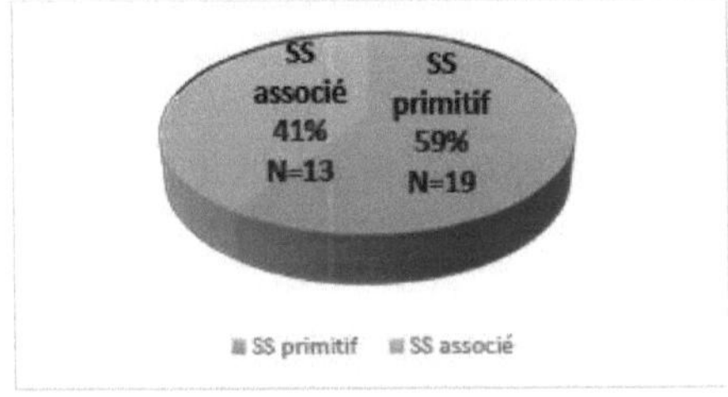

■ Primary SS BSS associates

Figure 9: Distribution of patients according to whether they had primary or associated Sjogren's syndrome.

113. Former :

The age of the xerostomy, calculated from the year of onset of symptoms, is shown in Figure 10.

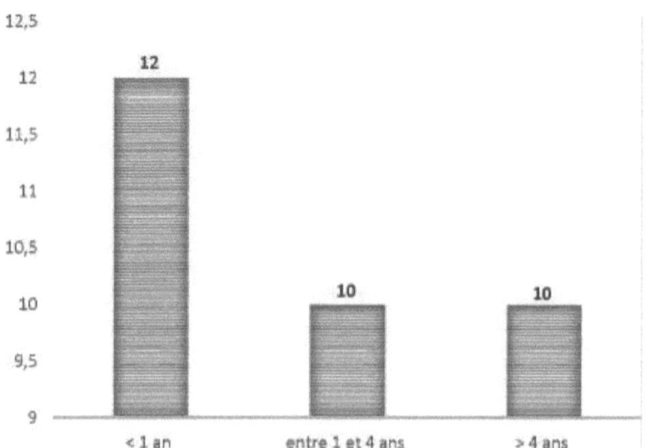

Figure 10: Number of patients by age of Sjogren's syndrome.

114. Glandular manifestations :

114.1. Oral manifestations :

114.1.1. Xerostomy :

As an inclusion criterion, dry mouth was present in all patients.

The characteristics of the patients' xerostomies are detailed in Table VI.

Table VI: Characteristics of the xerostomy at inclusion.

Symptom	Number of patients	Percentage
Sensation of dry, pasty mouth	32	100
Repeated fluid intake with meals	29	90
Intolerance to spicy or acidic foods	29	90
Inability to eat dry food	23	71
Gene during the speech	19	59
Dysphagia	19	59
Chronic burns of the oral mucosa	17	53
Inability to speak continuously	17	53
Food avoidance due to mouth pain	16	50
Dysgeusia	12	37
Gastro-resophageal reflux	4	12

114.1.2. Examination of the oral cavity :

Only one patient had dentures.

The abnormalities found on examination of the patients' oral cavity are detailed in Table VII.

Table VII: Examination of the oral cavity.

Symptom	Number of patients	Percentage

18

	Number of patients	Percentage
Cheilitis at the corners of the mouth	32	100
Dry, sticky oral mucosa	30	93
Dental caries	28	87
Erythema of the tongue	27	84
Cracks in the dorsal surface of the tongue	25	78
Papillary atrophy	24	75
Generalized erythema of the oral mucosa	19	59
Tooth lift	16	50
Erythema as a geographic map of the oral mucosa	4	12
Oral candidiasis	3	9
Salivary gland tumour	1	3

114.1.3. Biopsy of the accessory salivary glands :

Thirty-one patients underwent biopsy of the accessory salivary glands. Two biopsies were non-contributory.

The proportion of Chisholm grade 3 or 4 lymphocytic sialadenitis is shown in Figure 11.

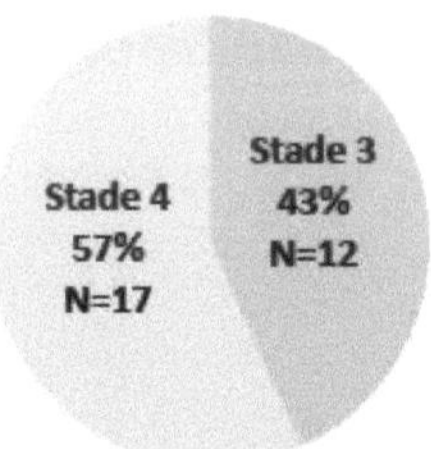

Figure 11: Proportion of lymphocytic sialadenitis on biopsy of the accessory salivary glands.

114.1.4. Other oral examinations :

Two patients underwent salivary scintigraphy, both of which showed hypofunction of the four salivary glands.

A parotid MRI scan carried out on one patient revealed an inflammatory aspect to the parotid glands.

114.2. Ocular manifestations :

114.2.1. Xerophthalmia :

Twenty-eight patients had xerophthalmia.

The various ocular symptoms are detailed in Table VIII.

Table VIII: Ocular symptoms.

Symptoms	Number of patients	Percentage
Dry eyes	28	87
Pruritus	23	74
Impression of a foreign body in the eyes	20	62
Burning sensation	20	62

Irritation	18	56
Photophobia	14	43

114.2.2. Ophthalmological examination :

All patients had at least one ophthalmological examination.

All patients had a break-up time. Thirty-one patients had a Schirmer test.

Thirty-one patients had at least one abnormality on ophthalmological examination. No patient had a corneal ulcer, keratitis or cecitis.

Ophthalmological abnormalities are detailed in Table IX.

Table IX: Ocular damage.

Ophthalmological examination	Number of patients	Percentage
Keratoconjunctivitis sicca	8	25
Mucin deposition in conjunctival cul-de-sacs	5	15
Decreased visual acuity	3	9
Break-up time	31	97
Schirmer test	28	87

114.3. Other glandular manifestations :

Fifty-nine per cent of patients had cutaneous dryness. The distribution of glandular skin, digestive, gynaecological and upper airway manifestations is shown in Figure 12.

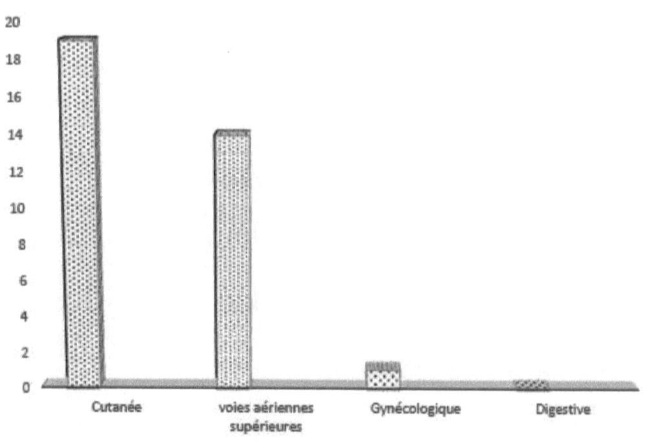

Figure 12: Distribution of glandular manifestations apart from xerophthalmia and xerostomy.

115. Extra-glandular manifestations :

The main extra-glandular manifestations diagnosed are shown in Figure 13.

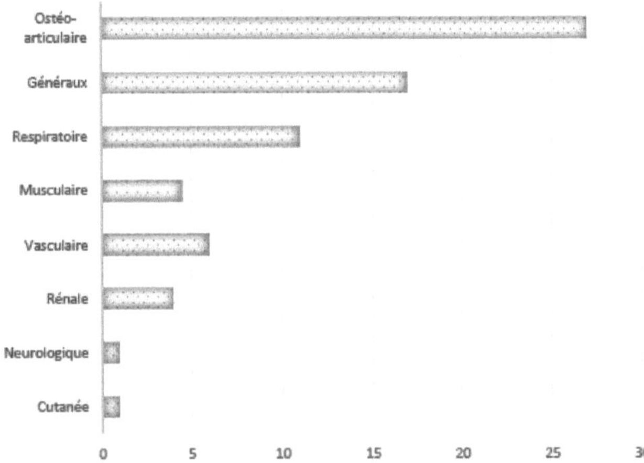

Figure 13: Distribution of extra-glandular manifestations.

Osteoarticular manifestations were represented by arthralgia (n=27) and arthritis (n=4). Respiratory symptoms included diffuse interstitial lung disease (n=6), isolated cough (n=4) and constrictive bronchiolitis (n=1).
The renal manifestations were represented by tubulo-interstitial damage in all 4 cases.
Seven patients had isolated myolysis without muscle deficit.
General signs included asthenia (n=16), fatigue (n=15) and weight loss (n=4).
Seven patients had Raynaud's syndrome. One patient had Waldenstom's hypergammaglobulinemic purpura.

116. Lymphoma :

None of the patients had lymphoma.

117. Immunoassay :

Thirty patients had positive antinuclear antibodies.
The immunological profile of the patients is shown in Figure 14.

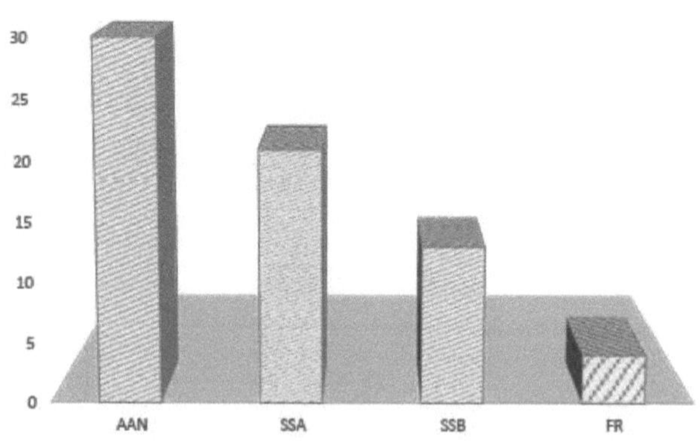

Figure 14: Immunological profile of patients.

Antinuclear antibodies were not found in six cases.

118. Treatment of Sjogren's syndrome :

Thirty patients were receiving symptomatic treatment. Two patients received corticosteroid therapy at a dose of 1 mg/Kg/day, prescribed in both cases as part of the management of diffuse interstitial lung disease.

The different drugs are detailed in table X.

Table X: Drugs prescribed for the treatment of Sjogren's syndrome.

Medicines	Number of patients	Percentage
Artificial tears	24	75
Tear gel	24	75
Bromhexine	22	68
Simple analgesic	18	56
Low-dose corticoids	8	25
Anetholtrithione	2	6
High-dose corticoids	2	6
Pilocarpine	1	3
Immunosuppressant	1	3

None of the patients received cevimeline.

IV. Inclusion scores :

1. EULAR Sjogren's Syndrome Patient Reported Index :

1.1. Total score :

The mean ESSPRI score was 21.5 with extremes between 12 and 30. Twenty-three patients (71.8%) had an ESSPRI score above 20. The distribution of patients according to the severity of the ESSPRI score is shown in Figure 15.

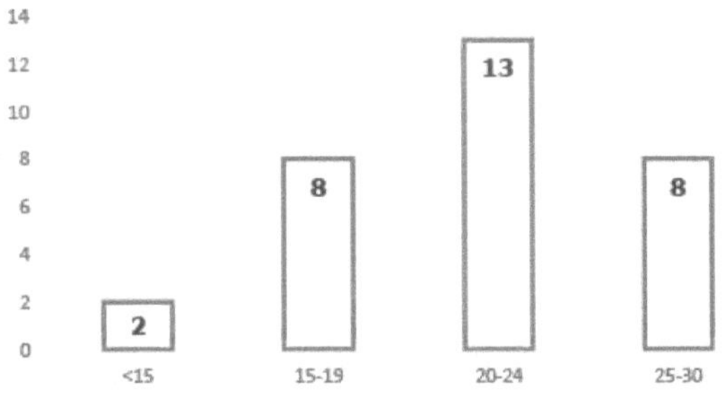

Figure 15: Distribution of patients according to severity of ESSPRI score.

1.2. Dry mouth:

No patient had an oral dryness score of less than 5. The mean dryness score was 7.41, with extremes between 5 and 10.

Fifty per cent of participants (n=16) had a dry mouth score of 8 or more. The distribution of patients according to the severity of oral dryness is shown in Figure 16.

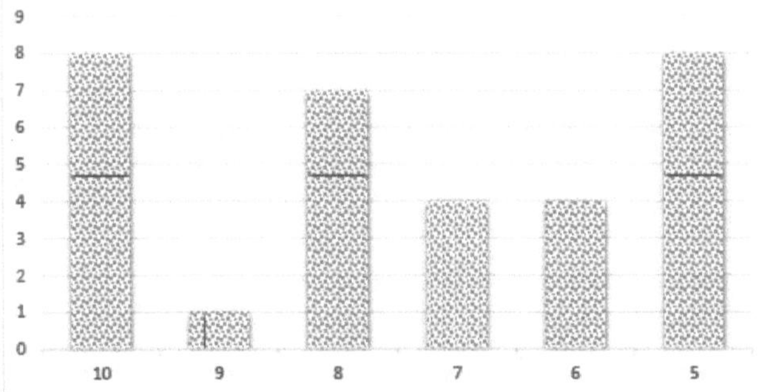

Figure 16: Distribution of patients according to the severity score for dry mouth.Fatigue :

The mean fatigue score was 7.72, with extremes between 2 and 10. Fifty-six per cent of patients had a score of 8 or more. The distribution of patients according to the severity of fatigue is shown in Figure 17.

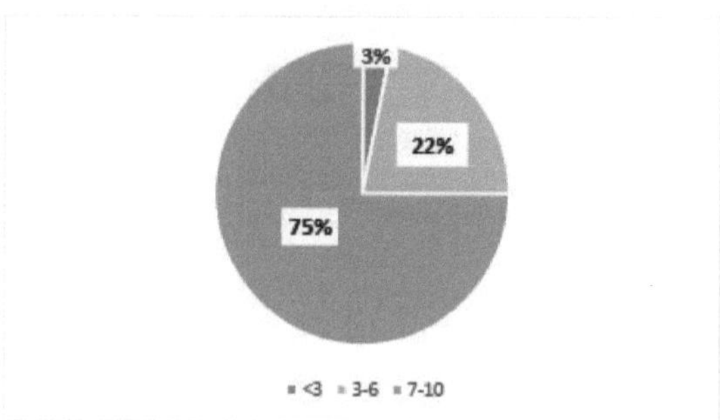

Figure 17: Distribution of patients according to fatigue score.

1.3. Pain :

Thirty-seven per cent of patients had a pain score of 8 or above. The mean pain score was 6.3 with extremes from 0 to 10.

The distribution of patients according to pain score is shown in Figure 18.

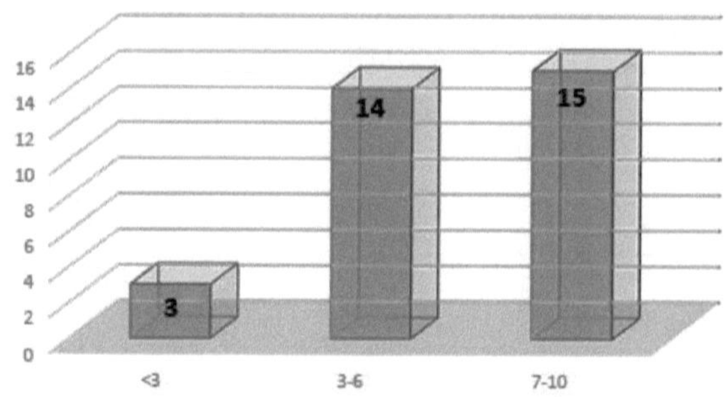

Figure 18: Distribution of patients according to pain score.

2. Xerostomia Inventory :

The mean Xerostomia Inventory score was 42.5 points out of 55, with extremes between 22 and 55. Forty-seven per cent of patients had a score above 45. The distribution of patients according to the severity of the Xerostomia Inventory score is shown in Figure 19.

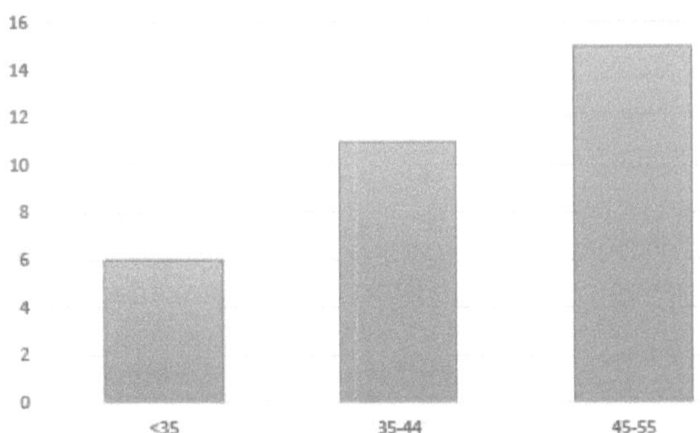

Figure 19: Distribution according to severity of the Xerostomia Inventory score.

3. Visual analogue scale :

The mean VAS score was 5.5 with extremes from 0 to 10. Ten patients or 31% of participants had a score greater than or equal to 7. The VAS score for global activity according to the patient's assessment is detailed in figure 20.

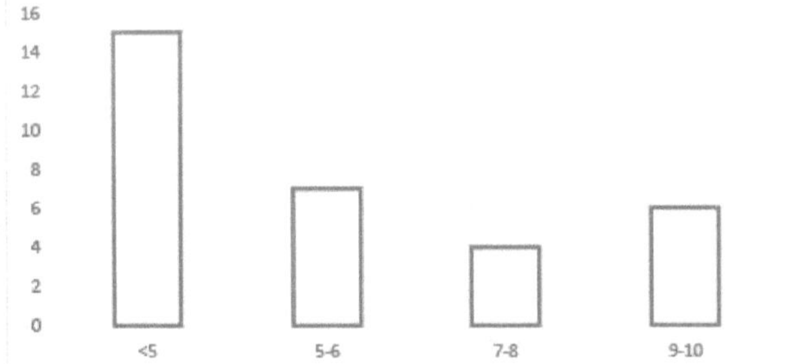

Figure 20: Distribution of patients according to VAS severity.

V. Assessment under usual treatment alone :

1. EULAR Sjogren's Syndrome Patient Reported Index :

1.1. Dry mouth:

The oral dryness response of patients on usual treatment alone in the 2 arms of the study is detailed in Table XI.

Table XI: Response of patients on usual treatment alone to dryness according to ESSPRI.

	Number of patients	Percentage
No improvement	3094	
Significant improvement		26 %

1.2. Fatigue :

The mean fatigue score under usual treatment was 7.59.

The response concerning fatigue in patients on usual treatment alone is detailed in Table XII.

Table XII: Response of patients on usual treatment alone to fatigue according to ESSPRI.

	Number of patients	Percentage
No improvement	31	97 %
Significant improvement	1	3 %

1.3. Pain :

The mean pain score under usual treatment was 6.62.

The response concerning pain in patients on usual treatment alone is detailed in Table XIII.

Table XIII: Response of patients on usual treatment alone to pain according to ESSPRI.

	Number of patients	Percentage
No improvement	30	94%
Significant improvement	2	6%

2. Xerostomia inventory :

Table XIV details the response of patients on usual treatment alone according to the Xerostomia Inventory score.

Table XIV: Responses of patients on usual treatment alone according to Xerostomia Inventory.

	Number of patients	Percentage
No improvement	30	94 %
Significant improvement	2	6 %

3. Visual analogue scale :

The mean VAS under usual treatment alone was 5.2.

Response to usual treatment alone, assessed by VAS score, is shown in Table XV.

Table XV: VAS score under usual treatment alone.

	Number of patients	Percentage
No improvement	31	97 %
Significant improvement	1	3 %

4. Examination of the oral cavity :

Table XVI shows the responses under usual treatment alone.

Table XVI: Oral cavity examination under usual treatment alone.

	Number of patients	Improvement	Percentage
Cheilitis at the corners of the mouth	32	3	9 %
Dry, sticky mucous membrane	30	2	6 %
Erythema of the tongue	27	1	3 %
Fissure on the dorsal surface of the tongue	25	0	-
Papillary atrophy	24	0	-
Generalized erythema of the oral mucosa	19	1	-

VI. Evaluation under olive oil mouthwash :

During the course of the study, 2 patients (6%) were excluded from the study protocol at 3^{dme} contact, i.e. at 6 weeks in randomised group B. Results are expressed on an intention-to-treat basis for a total of 32 patients.

1. EULAR Sjogren's Syndrome Patient Reported Index :

1.1. Dry mouth:

Table XVII shows the frequency of patient improvement with HO mouthwashes.

Table XVII: Oral dryness under olive oil according to ESSPRI.

Number of patients Percentage No improvement

1341 %

Significant improvement

1753 %

1.2. Fatigue :

The mean fatigue score for HO and usual treatment was 7.5.

Table XVIII details the response of patients taking olive oil to fatigue according to the ESSPRI score.

Table XVIII: Fatigue under olive oil according to ESSPRI.

	Number of patients	Percentage
No improvement	29	91 %
Significant improvement	1	3 %

1.3. Pain :

The mean pain score under HO was 6.63.

Table XIX details the response of patients on olive oil to pain according to the ESSPRI score.

Table XIX: Pain under olive oil according to ESSPRI.

	Number of patients	Percentage
No improvement	28	88%
Significant improvement	2	6 %

2. Xerostomia inventory :

2.1. Total score :

Table XX details the improvement in dry mouth with olive oil as assessed by the Xerostomia Inventory score.

**Table XX: Dry mouth under olive oil
according to Xerostomia Inventory.**

Number of patients Percentage

No improvement

619%

Significant improvement

2475%

2.2. Mini-Xerostomia Inventory :

Figure 21 shows the cumulative variation in the scores of the different questions numbered 1 to 11 proposed by the Xerostomia Inventory score of respondent patients before and after the use of olive oil.

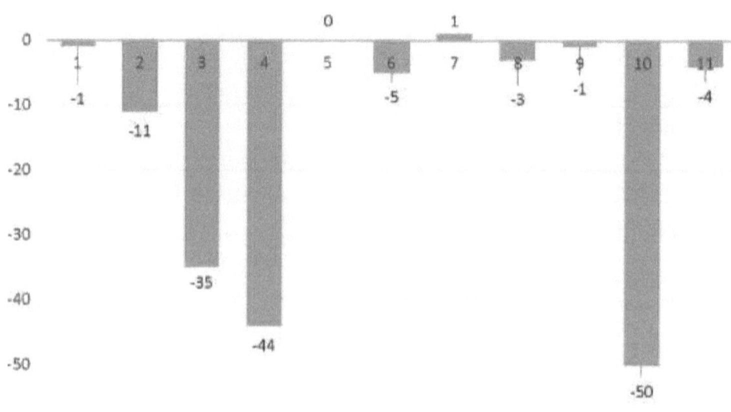

Figure 21: Variation in Xerostomia Inventory items in responders.

The 2eme , 3eme , 4eme and 10eme items (I feel a dry mouth when I eat, I wake up at night to drink water, I feel a dry mouth, My lips are dry) were combined to form the mini-Xerostomia Inventory.

The decrease in these four items (cumulative algebraic values) is greater than the rest of the questionnaire's proposals, with decreases of -11, -35, -44 and -50 for the 2eme , 3eme , 4eme and 10eme items respectively.

3. Visual Analogue Scale :

The mean VAS under HO was 4.9.

Table XXI shows the variation in response assessed by the VAS.

Table XXI: EVA score for olive oil.

	Number of patients	Percentage
No improvement	26	81 %
Significant improvement	4	12

4. Examination of the oral cavity :

Table XXII shows the significant responses under olive oil treatment.

Table XXII: Oral cavity examination under olive oil.

	Number of patients	Improvement	Percentage
Cheilitis at the corners of the mouth	32	26	81%
Dry, sticky mucous membrane	30	19	63%
Erythema of the tongue	27	24	75%
Fissure on the dorsal surface of the tongue	25	12	48%
Papillary atrophy	24	7	29%
Generalized erythema of the oral mucosa	19	15	-

5. Desire to continue treatment:

Twenty-eight patients wished to continue treatment with HO mouthwashes.

6. Undesirable effects of olive oil :

No undesirable effects were observed during the study.

B/ Analytical study :

I. Characteristics of the study population at inclusion :

Tables XXIII, XXIV and XXV show the distribution of age, gender and scores used at inclusion according to randomisation.

Table XXIII: Average age according to randomisation.

	Number of patients	Average age (years)	P
HO in V[re] period	16	52.25	NS
HO in 2®[me] period	16	51	

Table XXIV: Gender distribution according to randomisation.

			HO in V[re] period	HO in 2®[me] period	P
Type	Female	Workforce	14	15	NS
		Percentage	88%	94%	
	Male	Workforce	2	1	
		Percentage	12%	6%	

Table XXV: Distribution of ESSPRI, Xerostomia Inventory and EVA scores according to randomisation.

		Average	p
ESSPRI	HO in 1[idre] period	7,94	
	HO in 2[idme] periods	6,88	NS
Xerostomia Inventory	HO in 1[idre] period	42,56	NS
	HO in 2[idme] periods	42,56	
EVA	HO in 1[idre] period	5,625	NS
	HO in 2[idme] periods	5,375	

II. Evaluation of the primary endpoint :

Xerostomy :

1. EULAR Sjogren's Syndrome Patient Reported Index :

The improvement in the ESSPRI score under HO was greater than under usual treatment alone, with a significant difference (p<0.001).

Table XXVI details the distribution of responses under HO and usual treatment alone according to the ESSPRI score.

Table XXVI: Responses assessed by the ESSPRI score.

	Olive oil	Usual treatment alone	P
Improvement	172		
			<0.0001
No improvement	1328		

According to the ESSPRI score :
-    Patients who improved on HO (n=17) did not improve on usual treatment alone.
-    Patients who improved on usual treatment alone (n=2) did not improve on HO.
-    No patient improved in either arm of the study.
-    Eleven patients did not improve on either HO or standard treatment alone.

2. Xerostomia Inventory :

The improvement in the Xerostomia Inventory score under HO was greater than under usual treatment alone, with a significant difference (p<0.001).

Table XXVII details the distribution of responses under HO and under usual treatment alone according to the Xerostomia Inventory score.

Table XXVII: Responses assessed by the Xerostomia Inventory score.

	Olive oil	Usual treatment alone	P
Improvement	24	2	<0.001
No improvement	6	28	

According to the xerostomia inventory score :
-    Twenty-three patients improved on HO and did not improve on usual treatment alone.
-    One patient improved both on the usual treatment alone and on HO.
-    One patient improved on usual treatment alone and did not improve on HO.
-    Five patients did not improve on either HO or standard treatment alone.

III. Evaluation of secondary endpoints :

1. Visual analogue scale :

The improvement in VAS was not significant.

Table XXXX details the results obtained with HO and usual treatment alone.

Table XXXX: Responder patients assessed by VAS score. Olive oilUsual treatment alone p

	Olive oil	Usual treatment alone	p
Improvement	4	1	NS
No improvement	26	29	

According to the VAS score :
-    One patient improved on usual treatment alone and did not improve on olive oil.
-    Four patients improved with olive oil and did not improve with usual treatment alone.
-    Twenty-five patients improved neither with olive oil nor with the usual treatment alone.
-    No patient improved in either arm of the study.

2. Examination of the oral cavity :

The oral cavity abnormalities significantly improved under HO were dryness of the oral mucosa, tongue erythema and cheilitis of the labial commissures.

The improvement in these three criteria was not influenced by the primary or associated nature of the SS, randomisation, the month of application of the HO, the ESSPRI and Xerostomia Inventory scores at inclusion, or the age of the SS.

IV. **Parameters influencing the response to olive oil :**

1. Randomisation :

The distribution of ^amelioration of response under HO assessed by the ESSPRI and the Xerostomia Inventory according to randomisation is shown in Table XXVIII.

Table XXVIII: Responses under HO according to randomisation.

Score	Randomisation		TotalP	
	Olive oil in 1st period	Olive oil in 2nd period		
Improvement ESSPRI	10	7	17	NS
Amelioration Xerostomia Inventory	13	11	24	NS

2. Month of application :

The therapeutic responses assessed by the ESSPRI score and the Xerostomia Inventory score according to the months during which olive oil was used are detailed in Table XXIX.

Table XXIX: Response under olive oil according to the month of application of olive oil.

score	Month		TotalP	
	January to March	April to June		
Improvement ESSPRI5		12	17	NS
Xerostomia improvement9 Inventory		15	24	NS

3. Former :

Table XXX shows the distribution of patients with an improvement under HO as assessed by the ESSPRI score and the Xerostomia Inventory score, according to the age of SS.

Table XXX: Response to olive oil according to the age of Sjogren's syndrome.

score	Old		Total	P
	< 3 years	>3 years		
Improvement ESSPRI6		11	17	NS
Amelioration Xerostomia Inventory8		16	24	NS

4. Primitive or associated :

Table XXXI shows the improvement under HO as assessed by the ESSPRI score and the Xerostomia Inventory score, depending on whether the SS was primary or associated.

Table XXXI: Responses under olive oil according to the primary or associated nature of the SS.

Score	Sjogren's syndrome		Total	P
	Primitive	Associate		

Improvement ESSPRI [11]	6	17	NS
Amelioration Xerostomia Inventory [16]	8	24	NS

5. ESSPRI score at inclusion :

Table XXXII shows the distribution of significant responses to olive oil as assessed by the ESSPRI score and the Xerostomia Inventory score according to the ESSPRI score at inclusion.

Table XXXII: Response to olive oil according to ESSPRI score at inclusion.

Score	ESSPRI a l'inclusion		Total	P
	<8	>8		
Improvement ESSPRI	6	11	17	NS
Amelioration Xerostomia Inventory [11]	13	24	NS

6. Xerostomia Inventory score at inclusion :

The response to olive oil as assessed by the ESSPRI and the XI according to the Xerostomia Inventory score at inclusion is shown in Table XXXIII.

Table XXXIII: Response to olive oil according to the Xerostomia Inventory score at inclusion.

Score	XI a l'inclusion		Total	P
	<35	>35		
Improvement ESSPRI	5	12	17	NS
Amelioration Xerostomia Inventory [6]	18	24	NS

7. Extra-glandular manifestations :

Table XXXIV shows the distribution of patients who improved with olive oil, as assessed by the ESSPRI score and the Xerostomia Inventory score, according to whether or not they had joint damage.

Table XXXIV: Response to olive oil according to joint damage.

Score	Joint damage		P
	yes	No	
Improvement ESSPRI	15	2	NS
Amelioration Xerostomia Inventory [20]	4	NS

As regards the other extra-glandular disorders collected during the study (general signs (n=17), pulmonary (n=11), muscular (n=7), vascular (n=7), renal (n=4) and neurological (n=1) disorders, the number of patients did not allow statistical calculation.

8. Immunoassay :

Table XXXV shows the distribution of significant responses under HO as assessed by the

ESSPRI score and the Xerostomia Inventory score, depending on whether or not the immunological test was positive.

The immunological work-up was considered positive if the patient had a significant level of positive anti-nuclear antibodies and/or antibodies to SSA +/- SSB and/or Ro52.

Table XXXV: Response to olive oil according to immunological assessment.

Score	Immunological tests		P
	Positive	Negative	
Improvement ESSPRI	16	1	NS
Amelioration Xerostomia Inventory	22	2	NS

9. Treatment of xerostomia :

The distribution of ^amelioration of ESSPRI and xerostomia inventory scores under olive oil according to bromhexine intake is shown in Table XXXVI.

Table XXXVI: Response to olive oil according to bromhexine intake.

Score	Bromhexine		P
	Yes	No	
Improvement ESSPRI	9	8	NS
Xerostomia improvement Inventory	13	11	NS

Two patients were receiving anetholtritone, 1 of whom improved significantly according to the ESSPRI score and 1 of whom did not improve according to the ESSPRI and Xerostomia Inventory scores.

A patient being treated with pilocarpine improved significantly on olive oil according to both the ESSPRI and Xerostomia Inventory scores.

10. Fatigue :

Table XXXVII shows the distribution of the improvement in ESSPRI and Xerostomia Inventory scores with olive oil according to the degree of fatigue.

Fatigue was considered significant from a score of 7 or more out of 10.

Table XXXVII: Response to olive oil according to severity of fatigue.

Score	Significant fatigue		p
	Yes	No	
Improvement ESSPRI	12	5	NS
Xerostomia improvement Inventory	18	6	NS

11. Pain :

Table XXXVIII shows the distribution of the improvement in ESSPRI and Xerostomia Inventory scores under olive oil according to the degree of pain.

Pain was considered significant when the score was greater than or equal to 7 out of 10.

Table XXXVIII: Response to olive oil according to the degree of pain.

Score	Severe pain		p
	Yes	No	
Improvement ESSPRI	8	9	NS
Amelioration Xerostomia Inventory	10	14	NS

12. Visual Analogue Scale :

Table XXXIX shows the distribution of the improvement in ESSPRI and Xerostomia Inventory scores under olive oil according to the VAS at inclusion.

The EVA score was considered high if it was greater than or equal to 7 out of 10.

Table XXXIX: Response under olive oil according to EVA.

Score	High EVA		p
	Yes	No	
Improvement ESSPRI	4	13	NS
Amelioration Xerostomia Inventory	8	16	NS

4 DISCUSSION

The HOSS study was conducted in patients with primary or associated Sjogren's syndrome. It was a prospective, randomised, single-blind crossover study. The aim of the study was to evaluate the effect of HO mouthwash on xerostomia. Patients were randomised into 2 groups. Patients randomised to group A received HO in the first[re] period (the first 3 weeks) and their usual treatment alone in the second[eme] period (the last 3 weeks). The periods were reversed in the event of randomisation to group B. Xerostomia was assessed by ESSPRI and Xerostomia Inventory scores. A global evaluation of the disease using the VAS, a search for associated glandular and extra-glandular manifestations and an examination of the oral cavity were carried out. All these assessments were repeated on 3 occasions (at inclusion, 3 weeks and 6 weeks).

At the end of the 6-month study, 32 patients were included. The epidemiological characteristics of the patients corresponded to the profile of patients with Sjogren's syndrome, with an average age of 51.6 years and a gender ratio of 1:10.

The results of our study showed a significant improvement in xerostomia with olive oil mouthwashes in 53% of patients according to the ESSPRI score and 75% according to the Xerostomia Inventory score, with a significant difference compared with usual treatment alone.

No studies have looked at HO as a treatment for xerostomia. The results of our study will be compared with other therapies.

I. Limitations and biases of the study :

1. Randomisation :

The simple randomisation of patients using a pre-established table at the time of treatment allocation helped to reduce selection bias. It is certainly true that more complex computerised randomisation tables are available. These allow a distribution that cannot be predicted by the doctor. However, simple randomisation is accessible without specific software and remains just as valid [16].

2. Number of patients :

The number of patients in our study was 32. This is not a very large number, but it is sufficient to meet our objectives. This number is greater than the number needed for theoretical calculations.

SS is an uncommon disease, with a prevalence in France of between 0.1 and 0.4% of the adult population and an incidence of around 4 to 5 new cases per 100,000 population. This makes it a rare disease [1]. We have no prevalence or incidence figures for Sjogren's syndrome in Tunisia. Nevertheless, a multicentre study conducted under the aegis of the Tunisian Society of Internal Medicine collected 112 cases of Sjogren's syndrome in 9 internal medicine departments between 1990 and 2002.

Furthermore, in the absence of therapeutic modification, dry mouth was stable outside the first few months. Patients whose symptoms had been evolving for less than 6 months were not included.

3. Inclusion, non-inclusion and exclusion criteria :

Patients with other causes of dry mouth not included in the AECG 2002 exclusion criteria could have been excluded, such as patients with diabetes or systemic scleroderma... These pathologies could have affected the interpretation of the results.

However, in therapeutic trials of Sjogren's syndrome, these pathologies have not been excluded.

4. Cross shot :

In a crossover trial, the subject receives 2 or more treatments successively or simultaneously in random order. Each patient is matched to himself. The time a patient participates in the trial is divided into 2 periods. During each of these periods, the patient receives a different treatment.

Two treatment sequences are possible: the treatment studied first, then the control treatment, or the control treatment first, then the treatment studied.

The experimental cross-over design used is the most appropriate for this therapeutic trial. On the one hand, xerostomy in SS has a stable chronic course beyond the first few months during which oral dryness may worsen [1]. Patients with symptoms evolving for less than 6 months were not included.

On the other hand, the effect of olive oil is measurable in the short term.

Thus, the chronicity of the disease and the measurable nature of the short-term treatment effect make the crossover plan an ideal design for our study [17].

In addition, cross-over has made it possible to eliminate inter-individual variability. This is all the more important in Sjogren's syndrome, a systemic disorder with a protean clinical expression, which may be associated with other autoimmune diseases as part of an associated Sjogren's syndrome.

This type of matching ensures a high degree of comparability between the control and intervention groups, since the same patient passes through both groups. Only intra-individual variability remains.

The variance of the measurement of the treatment effect is thus reduced compared with a design with 2 parallel groups. Correlation between the measurements made on the same patient is a necessary condition for obtaining a reduction in variance with the cross-over design.

5. Wash out period:

A wash-out period can be arranged between the two periods. This period allows the treatment administered first to wear off, along with its effects.

In our study, HO was randomised into 1ere or 2eme periods with no washout period.

The results showed that response to treatment was not influenced by randomisation. This shows, on the one hand, that the period effect was counteracted and, on the other hand, that the effect of olive oil is suspensive and not curative. The absence of a washing period therefore did not affect the results of our study.

6. Duration of the study :

The study was spread over 6 months: from January to June. The correlation of the results according to the month of application of the HO showed no significant difference between patients who had applied the HO during the winter (from January to March) and those who had had it during the spring (between April and June).

The summer period was not included in the study, nor was the Ramadan period. These are periods during which xerostomia can worsen and the effectiveness of HO could have been reduced. In addition, the inclusion of the summer period could have influenced the comparability of the groups through a period effect.

7. Placebo :

No placebo was used. It was difficult to find a product that resembled HO in every way, making it identical to it. The colour and viscosity were accessible, but the smell and taste were inimitable. The therapeutic trial was conducted without a placebo, in the absence of a valid placebo.

However, a comparison with other oils could have been suggested (linseed oil, almond oil, corn oil, etc.).

8. Judging criteria :

The primary endpoint of our study was an improvement in oral dryness detected by the 1ere ESSPRI oral dryness question of 20% and/or a decrease in the Xerostomia Inventory score of at least 3 points. The primary endpoint of our study was subjective.

Increasing the number of subjective scores by using the ESSPRI and Xerostomia Inventory scores improved the quality of data collection at inclusion and follow-up.

Measurement of salivary flow (stimulated or unstimulated) has been used in several studies as a primary or secondary endpoint for local therapies (Aagaard 1992, Andersson 1995, Bots 2005) [18-21]. This examination is classically described as simple, reproducible and inexpensive. A number of precautions must be taken before it is performed. Patients should not smoke, brush their teeth, drink or eat for at least one hour before the examination. In a graduated beaker, the patient allows his saliva to flow for 5 minutes. The direct reading on the graduations of the cup gives an estimate of the saliva flow. Saliva flow can be stimulated by chewing or by bitter or acidic taste. Normal salivary flow is 0.25 to 0.35mL/mn at rest and 1 to 2mL/mn after stimulation. This assessment reflects the quantitative alteration of saliva.

From a practical point of view, saliva flow is less straightforward. Firstly, letting the saliva flow seems simple, but patients tend to spit or swallow some of the saliva, even if they don't want to. This can lead to inter- and intra-individual variability, independent of the treatment.

Furthermore, the alteration in saliva production in Sjogren's syndrome is both quantitative and qualitative. This is supported by the fact that the functional gene is not necessarily correlated with salivary flow. A satisfactory salivary flow for one patient may be troublesome for another and vice versa. It is therefore recommended to treat a xerostomy even in the presence of normal salivary flow [21].

9. Olive oil of choice :

The olive oil chosen is a Tunisian extra-virgin oil available on the international market, sold in an opaque glass bottle.

The sample used for the chemical analysis of the olive oil was taken from a bottle of commercial olive oil. The various components of the selected olive oil are detailed in the appendix. The study of the chemical characteristics concluded that the olive oil was virgin.

The difference between a virgin olive oil and an extra-virgin olive oil is based essentially on 3 characteristics: acidity level, peroxide value and sensory analysis [23]. The acidity level and peroxide value of the sample supplied to the National Oil Board corresponded to the levels for extra-virgin olive oil. However, the sensory analysis concluded that it was virgin olive oil. This discrepancy may be due to the 30 days that elapsed before the oil sample delivered to the laboratory was analysed.

The grade of olive oil may be affected by environmental factors. The oil should be kept away from light and at a temperature as close as possible to 15°C. To avoid rancidity, the oil should not be in direct contact with the air.

The change in the character of olive oil from extra-virgin to virgin leads us to discuss 2 important points. The first is that patients may not have received the same quality of oil, given the importance of environmental factors and the storage conditions of the oil sample. This correlation cannot be verified a posteriori. Furthermore, it is not practically feasible to check the quality of the oil each time it is used, as this would require systematic analysis of every sample taken before and after use. This leads us to the 2[eme] important point, which is to stress to patients the importance of storing the oil away from light and heat, and also the importance of buying small bottles of olive oil to reduce contact with the air.

II. Effects of olive oil as a mouthwash:

The results of our study showed a significant improvement in xerostomia with olive oil mouthwashes in 53% of patients according to the ESSPRI score and 75% according to the Xerostomia Inventory score, with a significant difference compared with the usual treatment alone. The hypothesis formulated was thus confirmed.

Several parameters confirm that the improvement observed is indeed due to the effect of the application of HO and not to chance or a placebo effect. Firstly, this improvement is far greater than the 30% improvement in the case of a placebo effect [24].

In addition, the ESSPRI pain and fatigue scores remained stable under HO and usual treatment alone. This supports the fact that the improvement in oral dryness scores was due to the treatment and not to a placebo effect or chance.

In addition, the Xerostomia Inventory score contains 11 questions. Four of these are directly related to xerostomia, which we considered in the previous chapter as a Mini-Xerostomia Inventory. The decrease in the Mini-Xerostomia Inventory is superimposable on the total decrease in the Xerostomia Inventory score. This proves that the variation of the score is secondary to the improvement of the xerostomy and not to the other items such as skin dryness, dysphagia, xerorhinia and xerophthalmia.

The results showed a greater percentage improvement in the Xerostomia Inventory than in the ESSPRI, with 75 and 53% of patients respectively. Eight patients in whom the ESSPRI score did not improve had a significant decrease in the Xerostomia Inventory score.

This difference could be explained by the number of questions contained in each questionnaire. The ESSPRI score contains a single global question on dry mouth, whereas the Xerostomia Inventory explores the different aspects of xerostomia in greater detail and provides severity ratings.

In addition, this discrepancy may be explained by the difficulty patients have in expressing their complaints in figures. The ESSPRI score uses numbers, whereas the Xerostomia Inventory uses words. It is easier for patients to translate their complaints into words. This gene was palpable during the various interviews. Several patients asked us to remind them of the number they had been given at the previous consultation in order to give them a higher or lower score, depending on whether they felt the situation had improved or worsened. This information was not communicated to the patient.

Examination of the oral cavity showed a significant improvement in cheilitis of the labial commissures, erythema and dryness of the oral mucosa under HO.

III. Pharmacological characteristics of olive oil :

The positive results of our study could be explained by the different pharmacological characteristics of olive oil.

Externally, olive oil has emollient and softening properties. Its lubricating action on mucous membranes and skin helps to improve dry mouth and hairiness [7].

Taste is an important oral salivary stimulus in the physiology of salivary secretion. Olive oil, being rich in flavours, represents an important salivary stimulus. Moreover, the bitter taste in particular provokes reflex hypersialorrhea. This bitterness is even more pronounced if the olives were picked early [25].

HO has anti-inflammatory properties. Oleocanthal, the main component of olive oil, has ibuprofen-like activity. Oleocanthal can inhibit cyclooxygenase through its anti-COX-1 and anti-COX-2 activity [26].

A study carried out in stable coronary patients showed that regular daily consumption of 50 ml of refined olive oil for 2 periods of 3 weeks preceded by 2 weeks of wash-out reduced biomarkers of inflammation such as IL-6 and CRP. The phenolic compounds in olive oil have been shown to reduce certain inflammatory mediators such as IL-6, TNF alpha, IL-1 beta and PGE2 [27,28].

Two clinical studies showed a significant drop in plasma concentrations of thromboxane B2 and leukotrienes B4 in healthy or dyslipidemic subjects who regularly consumed olive oil. This reduction was more marked in subjects consuming extra-virgin olive oil [29,30].

HO has an antioxidant action via a number of components, including tocopherols (vitamin E), phenolic compounds (tyrosol and hydroxytyrosol), seco-iridoids (oleuropein, demethyleuropein and ligstroside), carotenoids (betacarotene) and lignans (acetoxypinoresinol and pinoresinol), which have antioxidant activity both in vitro and in vivo [31-38].

This richness in antioxidants is explained by the fact that the fruit is exposed to the air and must therefore defend itself against oxygen. Virgin olive oil, which has undergone no refining or industrial treatment, is particularly rich in antioxidants.

Olive oil, with its emollient, anti-inflammatory and anti-oxidant properties, has been shown to improve xerostomy in patients with Sjogren's syndrome.

The response assessed by ESSPRI and Xerostomia Inventory on olive oil was not influenced by primary or secondary Sjogren's syndrome, month of olive oil application, severity of xerostomia, immunological profile, treatment, fatigue, pain or VAS score at inclusion. There was no correlation between response to treatment and other extra-glandular conditions.

This means that olive oil can be used in all patients with Sjogren's syndrome, whether primary or secondary, regardless of the severity of the xerostomy and other clinical manifestations of the disease, all year round.

IV. Comparison of olive oil as a mouthwash with other local treatments:

Various local treatments for xerostomia have been studied, but the data were not sufficient to recommend one of the molecules or preparations.

Several presentations were tested: mouthwash, lozenge, gel, spray, chewing gum, mucoadhesive disc or mucosecretion systems.

The 1er published controlled trial of a treatment for xerostomia was that of Kestov et al [39] in 1981. The authors compared an artificial saliva containing 2% carboxymethylcellulose (CMC) with a placebo (glycerine + lemon) mouthwash. One hundred and forty-eight patients with SS were randomised into 2 parallel groups. After 12 days of application, xerostomia, frequency of use and desire to continue treatment were assessed. The data showed no benefit in terms of xerostomy improvement (21% of patients on CMC and 5% on glycerin) or desire to continue treatment.

In 1982, Donatsky et al [40] conducted a crossover study in 15 patients with SS. The patients were randomised into 3 groups: 2 groups using sprays and a placebo group (water). One spray contained CMC, sorbitol, glycerine, lemon, salt and preservatives. The 2eme spray had the same composition except for the CMC. The primary endpoint was xerostomy reduction and patient preference. The results showed that after 2 weeks of treatment, there was no difference between the 2 sprays regarding xerostomy. The spray containing CMC resulted in a non-significant reduction in xerostomia compared with placebo. However, patients preferred the spray containing CMC to the base spray.

Gravenmade [41] in 1993 compared 42 patients with SS using a mucin lozenge versus placebo in a randomised crossover study with a 2-week wash-out period. There was no significant difference between the products regarding xerostomy and the number of lozenges used. Patients preferred the mucin lozenge. It is important to note, however, that this study had a reverse sex ratio with respect to pathology (41 men and only one woman), which indicates a selection bias that hinders interpretation of the results obtained.

In 1996, Van der Reijden [42] carried out a crossover study of 43 patients with SS using 3 artificial saliva substitutes versus placebo. The 3 saliva substitutes containing either carbopol, xanthan or orthana were used for 1 week. In addition to subjective criteria (xerostomia by VAS, patient preference, desire to continue the allocated treatment), this study evaluated objective criteria (stimulated and non-stimulated salivary flow). No spray was effective.

Andersson [43] in 1995 compared the effect of linseed oil spray for 3 weeks versus CMC in a crossover trial involving 20 patients with xerostomia secondary to radiotherapy. Salivary flow was studied in addition to subjective criteria. The authors reported a better response when linseed oil was used, with a significant difference: improvement in xerostomia and reduction in dental plaque. In addition, patients preferred linseed oil to CMC with a significant difference.

Another team was interested in linseed oil. In 2001, Johansson [44] conducted a crossover therapeutic trial on 33 patients with SS, evaluating linseed oil mouthwash versus linseed oil combined with chlorhexidine. The mouthwashes were applied twice a day for 3 weeks with a 3-week wash-out period. The authors reported an improvement in xerostomia with the 2 products, as well as an improvement in elocution problems and burning sensation with linseed oil alone.

Other vegetable oils have also been studied:

Rapeseed oil was used in a crossover therapeutic trial in 2005 conducted by Momm's team [45]. One hundred and twenty-three patients with xerostomia secondary to radiotherapy were randomised to receive rapeseed oil, CMC spray, aloe vera gel or mucin spray for 4 weeks. The results showed an improvement under the 4 proposed products compared with baseline but with no significant difference between them.

Pilocarpine was used as a lozenge by Taweechaisupapong et al [46] in 2006. This was a placebo-controlled crossover trial in 33 patients who had undergone head and neck irradiation. Patients were seen on 4 occasions for 3 hours after taking a 3 or 5 mg pilocarpine tablet. A xerostomy VAS and salivary flow were performed. There was a significant improvement in dry mouth and saliva production. There was no significant difference in speech difficulty and oral pain.

Pilocarpine mouthwashes were studied against 0.9% saline for 4 weeks by Kim et al [47] in 2013. Sixty patients with a xerostomy of any etiology for 3 months were randomised into 2 groups. There was no significant difference between the 2 groups with regard to dry mouth, waking up at night to drink water or salivary flow.

The Xerostomia system ® oral care system consists of a toothpaste and mouthwash containing olive oil, betaine, xylitol, fluoride, vitamin E and vitamin B5. In a study conducted by Ship [48] in 2007, the Xerostomia system ® showed a significant improvement in xerostomia and thirst compared to usual treatment. However, patients with SS were excluded from this study.

There is therefore insufficient evidence to recommend any of these local treatments.

Table XXXX: Different local treatments for xerostomia.

Author Année	Kestov 1981	Donastsky 1982	Gravenmade 1993	Andersson 1995	Van der reijden 1996	Johanson 2001	Momni 2005	Taweechaisupapong 2006	Kim 2013	Our study HOSS
Molecule	CMC*	CMC*	Mucine	Linseed oil	Carbopol Xanthan Orthana	Linseed oil chlorhexidine	Rapeseed oil CMC/Aloe Vera/ Mucine	Pilocarpine	Pilocarpine	Olive oil
Presentation	Saliva artificial	Spray	Pastille	Spray	Saliva artificial	Mouthwash	Spray Gel	Pastille	Mouthwash	Mouthwash
N	148	15	42	20	43	33	123	33	60	32
SS+/Other	Yes/No	Yes/No	Yes/No	No/Yes	Yes/No	Yes/No	No/Yes	No/Yes	Yes/Yes	Yes/No
Type of study	Parallele	Parallele	Cross	Cross	Cross	Cross	Cross	Cross	Parallele	Cross
Duration (days)	12	14	14	21	7	21	28	10	28	21
Placebo	Yes	Yes	Yes	No	Yes	No	No	Yes	Yes	No
Randomisation	Yes	Yes	Yes	Yes	Yes	Yes	Yes	Yes	Yes	Yes
Wash-out	No	No	Yes	Yes	Yes	Yes	No	Yes	No	No
Judging criteria	Subjective	Subjective	Subjective	Subjective+ Objective	Subjective Objective	Subjective	Subjective	Subjective + Objective	Subjective+ Objective	Subjective

Improvem ent	Yes	Yes	Yes	Yes	No	Yes	Yes	Yes	Yes	Yes
Significant	No	No	No	Yes	No	No	No	Yes	No	Yes

V. Comparison of olive oil as a mouthwash versus oral treatments :

Oral pilocarpine and cevimeline are considered to be the two most effective drugs for the management of xerostomia in Sjogren's syndrome [49].

1. Efficiency :

1.1. Pilocarpine :

Oral pilocarpine has been shown to be effective against xerostomia.

Three hundred and seventy-three patients with a mean age of 55 years were randomised into 3 groups: pilocarpine 2.5mg 4 times/day (n=121), pilocarpine 5mg 4 times/day (n=127) and placebo (n=125) for 12 weeks [50]. The primary endpoint was the percentage of responders defined as having a VAS score between 55 and 100 mm for overall improvement in xerostomy and oral discomfort. Improvement in xerostomia with 20 mg pilocarpine was 63.1% and in oral discomfort 52.1% with a significant difference compared to placebo. There was no improvement in baseline salivary flow but a significant increase in salivary flow after 30, 60, and 90 minutes of taking 5 mg of pilocarpine.

Another study looked at pilocarpine. Two hundred and fifty-six patients with a mean age of 57 years were randomised into 2 groups: pilocarpine at a dose of 5 to 7.5mg 4 times/day (n=128) and placebo (n=128) [51]. The initial dose was 5mg 4 times/day for 6 weeks. This dose was increased to 7.5mg 4 times/day for the following 6 weeks. The overall improvement in xerostomia and discomfort was 57.4% and 60.7% respectively. Salivary flow measured at 60eme minutes post-dose was greater with pilocarpine than with placebo.

1.2. Cevimeline :

In 2002, Petrone et al [52] conducted a randomised controlled double-blind study of cevimeline versus placebo in 197 patients receiving 15 or 30 mg of cevimeline 3 times daily or placebo for 12 weeks. The primary endpoint was patient satisfaction with an "improved, stable or worsened" response. The secondary outcome was a VAS assessment of overall mouth sensation, dry mouth, dry tongue, ability to speak without drinking water, ability to chew and swallow food and sleep. Sixty-six per cent of patients had an improvement in xerostomia on cevimeline 90mg daily with a significant difference compared to placebo and the cevimeline 45mg daily group (45% improvement). The VAS assessment showed a significant improvement over placebo in the 90mg cevimeline daily group for overall mouth sensation, dry mouth and ability to speak without drinking.

Fife et al [53] conducted a randomised, placebo-controlled, double-blind study of cevimeline in 2002. Seventy-five patients with SS were enrolled and divided into 3 groups, each receiving 30mg cevimeline 3 times daily (n=25) or 60mg cevimeline 3 times daily (n=27) or placebo (n=23) for 6 weeks. The primary endpoint was improvement in xerostomia as judged by the patient as "improved, stable or worsened" and a VAS assessment of overall mouth sensation, mouth dryness, tongue dryness, ability to speak without drinking water, ability to chew and swallow food and sleep. There was an improvement in dry mouth sensation in 76% of patients taking 90mg cevimeline and 67% of patients taking 180mg cevimeline with a significant difference versus placebo. An improvement in overall mouthfeel, dry mouth and dry tongue with a significant difference compared to placebo.

■=> Our study showed that olive oil in mouthwash provides a response rate comparable to 20 mg pilocarpine and 90 mg cevimeline. The considerable advantage of HO as a mouthwash compared with these two molecules is the absence of adverse effects. However, a study comparing olive oil with pilocarpine and cevimeline needs to be carried out in order to better compare the efficacy and tolerance of these 3 molecules.

2. Tolerance :

2.1. Pilocarpine :

Out of 373 patients, 19 patients in the 10 mg pilocarpine group, 17 in the 20 mg pilocarpine group and 13 in the placebo group stopped treatment prematurely [50]. The adverse events encountered were: hypersudation (7.2% on placebo, 10.7% and 43.3% on 10 and 20 mg pilocarpine respectively), urinary frequency (1.6% on placebo, 10.7% and 9.5% on 10 and 20 mg pilocarpine respectively), vasomotor flushing (1.6% on placebo, 1.7% and 9.5% on 10 and 20 mg pilocarpine respectively).

In the second study evaluating pilocarpine, carried out on 256 patients, 19 of them stopped taking pilocarpine prematurely and 20 in the placebo group. Adverse events included hypersudation (64.1% versus 7% in the placebo group), urinary frequency (14.8% versus 5.5%), flushing (9.4% versus 3.1%) and chills (8.6% versus 0.8%). No deaths or serious treatment-related events have been reported [51].

These various undesirable effects are due to the pharmacodynamics of the compound. Its dose-dependent parasympathetic effect means that precautions must be taken in cases of asthma, cardiovascular disease, peptic ulcer, biliary lithiasis and underlying cognitive or psychiatric disorders.

Pilocarpine is contraindicated in patients with poorly controlled asthma, iridocyclitis, angle-closure glaucoma, pregnancy or breast-feeding. Precautions should also be taken in patients with impaired renal function or hepatic dysfunction.

2.2. Cevimeline :

Concerning cevimeline, in the study by Petrona et al [52] including 197 patients, 162 or 82.2% had at least one adverse event: 48.8% of patients taking 30mg cevimeline and 30.8% of patients taking 15mg. The most frequent events were nausea, hypersudation, abdominal pain and headache. These adverse events led to discontinuation of treatment in 16.1% of cases with cevimeline 30mg, 13.5% with 15mg and 4.3% with placebo.

In the study conducted by Fifa et al [53], 14 patients out of 75 withdrew from the study due to adverse drug reactions: 9 patients in the 60mg group, 4 in the 30mg group and 1 patient in the placebo group. All patients in the cevimeline 60mg group experienced at least one adverse event. The main complaints were hypersudation, nausea, headache, diarrhoea, vomiting and dizziness.

These undesirable effects remain a major limiting factor for these drugs, which are prescribed for patients whose quality of life is impaired by the disease itself. What's more, while waiting for a cure for SS, these symptomatic therapies are prescribed on a long-term basis. The undesirable effect is thus maintained by chronic use of the drug. The innocuousness of olive oil as a mouthwash is a considerable advantage, which supports its place in a long-term therapeutic plan. It is an everyday food product, widely acclaimed by nutritionists.

3. Cost and availability :

Another advantage of HO over pilocarpine and cevimeline is the cost of the product. Salagen® (pilocarpine) costs around 150 euros per month, or 370 Tunisian dinars per month. Evorax® (cevimeline) costs 178 dollars per month, or 392 Tunisian dinars per month. Olive oil mouthwash applied twice a day costs 3 Tunisian dinars a month. The large difference between the 2 reference molecules and HO is very attractive economically in times of crisis.

What's more, the availability of HO compared with pilocarpine and cevimeline makes it a serious competitor, especially in our country where the 2 molecules are not available.

VI. Chess :

In our study, xerostomia did not improve with olive oil mouthwashes in 6 patients. There were no significant epidemiological, clinical or immunological differences between patients who improved or did not improve with olive oil.

The quality of the oil was assessed by the national oil board as virgin and not extra virgin. This suggests that the patients may not have received the same quality of oil. This cannot be verified a posteriori.

Therapeutic compliance was judged to be good for all patients. However, an assessment of the quantity of oil used would have been a better reflection of compliance with mouthwash application.

Therapeutic modification may be suggested. One spoonful of HO was applied twice daily as a 5-minute mouthwash for 3 weeks. Patients who have not responded to this regimen may be offered an increase in the frequency, amount or duration of HO application. The abnormalities of the oral cavity that did not improve with olive oil mouthwashes were: fissures of the tongue (12/25), papillary atrophy (7/24) and dental caries (0/28). Tongue fissures and papillary atrophy are serious complications of dry mouth. Their management is difficult. Longer-term evaluation of olive oil is necessary. As far as cavities are concerned, the failure of olive oil as a mouthwash remains logical, as they can only be eradicated by dental treatment.

Fatigue and pain remained stable during the clinical trial. Olive oil as a topical treatment cannot act on these two components. The stability of these 2 components supports the objectivity of the responses provided by the patient and argues against a placebo effect.

There was no significant improvement in the VAS score assessing overall disease activity during our study, despite the improvement in xerostomy for some patients. This may be explained by the lack of improvement in the other systemic problems not affected by treatment, namely fatigue, pain and arthralgia. The lack of improvement in the ESSPRI score for fatigue and pain supports this hypothesis.

VII. Outlook:

We suggest using the equivalent of a teaspoon of HO as a mouthwash for at least 5 minutes, 2 or 3 times a day, combined with the application, using the amount taken from the teaspoon and the fingertip, of HO to the lips with the same frequency.

We recommend buying small opaque glass bottles of Tunisian extra-virgin HO. The bottles of HO should be kept away from heat. The importance of storing HO should be stressed to patients.

The improvement in oral dryness with an olive oil mouthwash leads us to consider other therapeutic perspectives.

Studies comparing the different types of Tunisian HO can be proposed in order to assess the effectiveness and tolerance of each of them.

A study by Creuzot's team [54] showed an improvement in xerophthalmia after regular consumption of polyunsaturated fatty acids, a compound rich in olive oil. This would make it possible to combine the consumption of olive oil with mouthwashes in order to act on xerophthalmia and xerostomia.

Experimental animal studies have shown that administration of a diet rich in olive oil reduces lymphocyte proliferation by inhibiting cytokine production and reducing Natural Killer activity. A therapeutic trial carried out on healthy volunteers showed that an infusion rich in olive oil emulsion for 6 hours reduced lymphocyte proliferation.

Another study showed that unsaturated fatty acids present in HO could modulate induced lymphoproliferation [55,56].

Animal studies suggest that a diet rich in olive oil reduces lymphocyte proliferation, inhibits cytokine production and reduces the activity of natural killer cells. This immunomodulatory activity is based in part on the unsaturated fatty acids contained in olive oil.

They are thought to reduce lymphoproliferation induced by mitogenes specific to B and T lymphocytes [57,58].

This immunomodulatory action could have an impact on the activity of a pathology whose pathophysiology is lymphoproliferation.

In addition, consumption of HO would therefore strengthen the immune system against attacks from micro-organisms. A study has shown that oleuropein has an immunomodulatory activity by promoting phagocytosis and inhibiting pro-inflammatory cytokines [59].

Several molecules studied, such as local pilocarpine and mucin pellets, were effective against xerostomia, whatever the etiology (ageing, drug-induced, post radiotherapy). Thanks to its safety and availability, the use of olive oil can be extended to other causes of xerostomia. However, further therapeutic trials are needed to assess the effect of HO on these different clinical situations.

5 CONCLUSIONS

Sjogren's syndrome is a systemic autoimmune disease whose clinical picture is dominated by a dry mouth and eye syndrome. The clinical manifestations of SS are multiple and vary in severity, but the dry syndrome remains the patient's main functional complaint. Local therapies are available but are not very effective. General therapies, in particular pilocarpine and cevimeline, are currently recommended but may have adverse effects and are not available in Tunisia. In the context of ancestral phytotherapy, some patients with SS have tried HO to relieve their dry mouth. This has led us to use HO as a local treatment for xerostomy in patients with Sjogren's syndrome.

The aim of the **HOSS** study was to evaluate the effect of Olive Oil mouthwash on xerostomia in patients with **Sjogren**'s Syndrome.

The hypothesis was that HO mouthwashes combined with the usual treatment significantly improved xerostomia in at least 40% of patients, with a significant difference compared with the usual treatment alone.

This was a prospective, randomised, single-blind, two-centre crossover study involving 32 patients with primary or associated Sjogren's syndrome evolving for more than 6 months, diagnosed according to the 2002 AECG criteria and with a xerostomy of 5 or more according to the ESSPRI score.

After giving their consent, patients were randomised into 2 groups. Patients randomised A received olive oil as a mouthwash in combination with their usual treatment in 1[iere] period and their usual treatment alone in 2[eme] period. The periods were reversed in case of randomisation B.

The olive oil chosen was a Tunisian extra-virgin oil available on the international market, sold in an opaque glass bottle. A sample was given to each participant in a 120 ml glass bottle. Each patient used the equivalent of one teaspoon of olive oil as a mouthwash for at least 5 minutes, twice a day, morning and evening, for 3 weeks. They also applied the same amount of HO to their lips with their fingertips at the same frequency as the teaspoon.

The primary endpoint of our study was an improvement in dry mouth detected by the 1[ere] ESSPRI question of 20% and/or a decrease in the Xerostomia Inventory score of at least 3 points.

The secondary endpoints were improvement in an abnormality found on examination of the oral cavity and a reduction in the VAS of 25 mm. These assessments were performed at inclusion, 3 weeks and 6 weeks by the same observer.

The results showed an improvement of the xerostomy in 17 patients according to the ESSPRI score and 26 patients according to the Xerostomia Inventory score, i.e. 53% and 75% of patients respectively, with a significant difference compared with the usual treatment alone. Examination of the oral cavity showed an improvement with a significant difference in cheilitis at the labial commissures, tongue erythema and dryness of the labial mucosa in 81%, 75% and 63% of patients respectively.

The limitations of our study are essentially represented by the absence of a placebo, the absence of a wash-out period and the non-inclusion of the summer period in the study. No placebo was valid because the smell and taste were unmistakable. The therapeutic trial was conducted without a placebo in the absence of a valid placebo. A wash-out period allowing the treatment administered first to disappear, along with its effects, could have been introduced between the two periods. However, the results showed that response to treatment was not influenced by randomisation. The absence of a washout period therefore did not affect the results of our study. The inclusion of the summer period could have influenced the comparability of the groups through a period effect. For this reason, the summer period was excluded.

The results enabled us to confirm the beneficial effect of olive oil as a mouthwash on xerostomia. This beneficial effect was independent of the primary or associated nature of the SS, the severity of the xerostomia, the month of application of the olive oil, the immunological profile, the treatment, fatigue, pain and the VAS score at inclusion. No correlation was found between response to treatment and other extra-glandular disorders.

The emollient and softening properties of olive oil explain the beneficial effect on xerostomia. The taste of olive oil directly stimulates salivary secretion.

Olive oil also has anti-inflammatory and anti-oxidant properties thanks to a number of components, including olecanthal, which has ibuprofen-like activity and can inhibit cyclooxygenase through its anti-COX-1 and anti-COX-2 activity, tocopherols, phenolic compounds, seco-iridoids, carotenoids and lignans, which have antioxidant activity both in vitro and in vivo.

During the course of the SS, other local therapeutics were studied: carboxymethylcellulose (CMC), mucin, carbopol, xanthan, orthana and pilocarpine. Vegetable oils such as linseed oil and rapeseed oil have been used as local treatments. Other more complex preparations were also evaluated. The most common presentations were mouthwashes, sprays, chewing gums and lozenges.

These studies were carried out in patients with Sjogren's syndrome or another cause of xerostomy, such as radiotherapy to the head and neck, or in elderly patients. However, there was insufficient data to recommend these local treatments, either because the improvement was not significant or because the number of patients was insufficient.

Oral pilocarpine and cevimeline are considered to be the two most effective molecules. The percentage improvement in xerostomia is around 60% for pilocarpine and 65% for cevimeline. However, the undesirable effects due to the pharmacological properties of the 2 molecules remain significant: sweating, abdominal pain, pollakiuria, vasomotor flushing, nausea, cephalea, etc.

Pilocarpine and cevimeline cost 150 euros (370 Tunisian dinars) and 178 dollars (392 Tunisian dinars) per month respectively. Furthermore, salagen® (pilocarpine) and evorax® (cevimeline) are not available in Tunisia.

Olive oil as a mouthwash gave a response rate comparable to 20 mg pilocarpine and 30 mg cevimeline. The considerable advantage of olive oil as a mouthwash over these two molecules is the absence of adverse effects. In addition, its availability and low cost make it a serious therapeutic alternative in a long-term project.

In our study, xerostomia did not improve with olive oil mouthwashes in 6 patients, with no difference from the clinical profile of patients who improved with olive oil. This failure may suggest poor compliance with therapy, which was denied by the patients. However, an assessment of the quantity of oil used would have been a better reflection of compliance with mouthwash application. The quality of the oil was assessed by the national oil board as virgin rather than extra virgin. This suggests that patients may not have received the same quality of oil depending on the storage and packaging conditions.

Patients who fail may be offered intensified therapy. An increase in the frequency, quantity or duration of HO may be proposed.

Tongue fissures, papillary atrophy and dental caries did not improve with olive oil mouthwash. More specific treatment is required.

Fatigue and pain remained stable during the clinical trial. Olive oil as a topical treatment cannot act on these two components. The lack of improvement in the VAS score assessing overall disease activity can be explained by the lack of improvement in other systemic conditions. This reinforces the results of our study by excluding the placebo effect.

Based on the results of our study, we suggest using the equivalent of a teaspoon of HO as a mouthwash for at least 5 minutes, 2 or 3 times a day, combined with the application of more HO to the lips with the same frequency, using the amount taken from the teaspoon and the fingertip.

We recommend buying small opaque glass bottles of Tunisian extra virgin OLIVE OIL. The bottles of HO should be kept away from heat. Patients should be made aware of the importance of storing HO.

The improvement in oral dryness with an olive oil mouthwash leads us to consider other therapeutic perspectives.

Regular consumption of polyunsaturated fatty acids rich in olive oil has been shown to improve xerophthalmia. This allows us to combine the consumption of olive oil with mouth rinses in order to act on xerophthalmia and xerostomia.

Experimental studies on animals have evaluated the benefits of a diet rich in olive oil. The results showed a reduction in lymphocyte proliferation with inhibition of cytokine production, a reduction in Natural Killer activity, a reduction in lymphocyte proliferation with an immunomodulatory action. Consumption of HO therefore helps to strengthen the immune system against attacks from micro-organisms.

In addition, several of the molecules studied were effective against xerostomia, whatever the etiology. Thanks to its safety, availability and low cost, the use of olive oil can be extended to other causes of xerostomia. However, further therapeutic trials are needed to assess the effect of olive oil in these different indications.

REFERENCES

1. Mariette X. Gougerot-Sjogren syndrome In: Guillevin L, Meyer O, Sibilia J, dir. Traite des maladies et syndromes systemiques. Paris: Flammarion Medecine- Sciences; 2008. P483-515.

2. Varoquier C, Salmon J, Sibilia J, Gottenberg J. Diagnostic criteria for Sjogren's syndrome. Rev Prat. 2012;62(2):225-8.

3. Vitali C, Bombardieri S, Jonsson R, Moutsopoulos H, Alexander E, Carsons S et al. Classification criteria for Sjogren's syndrome: a revised version of the European criteria proposed by the American-European Consensus Group. Ann Rheum Dis. 2002;60:554-8.

4. La Production [Online]. Office National de I'Huile [cited 02/06/2016] ; [about 3 screens]. Available at URL: http://www.onh.com.tn/index.php/fr/2016-05-23-14-44-46/la-production

5. Gigon F, Le Jeune R. Olive oil, Olea europaea L.. Phytotherapie. 2010;8:129-35.

6. Ghedira K. The olive tree. Phytotherapie. 2008;6:83-9.

7. Bruneton J. Pharmacognosie Phytochimie Plantes medicinales. 3eme edition. Paris: Technique et Documentation; 1999.

8. Breton C. Reconstruction de I'histoire de I'olivier (Olea europaea subsp. Europaea) et de son processus de domestication en region mediterraneenne, etudies sur des bases moleculaires [These]. Biologie des populations et ecologie: Aix-Marseille; 2006. 95p.

9. Gondouin A, Manzoni P, Ranfaing E, Brun J, Cadranel J, Sadoun D et al. Exogenous lipid pneumonia: a retrospective multicentre study of 44 cases in France. Eur Respir J. 1996;9(7):1463-9.

10. Alomirah H, Al-Zenki S, Husain A, Sawaya W, Ahmed N, Gevao B et al. Benzo[a]pyrene and total polycyclic aromatic hydrocarbons (PAHs) levels in vegetable oils and fats do not reflect the occurrence of the eight genotoxic PAHs. Food Addit Contam Part A Chem Anal Control Expo Risk Assess. 2010;27(6):869-78.

11. Rodnguez-Acuna R, del Carmen Perez-Camino M, Cert A, Moreda W. Polycyclic aromatic hydrocarbons in spanish olive oils: relationship between benzo(a)pyrene and total polycyclic aromatic hydrocarbon content. J Agric Food Chem. 2008;56(21):10428-32.

12. Bowman SJ, Booth DA, Platts RG, Field A, Rostron J, UK Sjogren's Interest Group. Validation of the Sicca symptoms Inventory for clinical studies of Sjogren's syndrome. J Rheumatol. 2003;30:1259-66.

13. Seror R, Theander E, Brun JG, Ramos-Casals M, Valim V, Dorner T et al. Validation of EULAR primary Sjogren's syndrome disease activity (ESSDAI) and patient indexes (ESSPRI). Ann Rheum Dis. 2015;74(5):859-66.

14. Thomson WM, Van der Putten GJ, de Baat C, Ikebe K, Matsuda K, Enoki K et al. Shortening the Xerostomia Inventory. Oral Surg Oral Med Oral Pathol Oral Radiol Endod. 2011;112(3):322-7.

15. Pai S, Ghezzi EM, Ship JA. Development of a Visual Analogue Scale questionnaire for subjective assessment of salivary dysfunction. Oral Surg Oral Med Oral Pathol Oral Radiol Endod. 2001;91:311-6.

16. Suresh KP. An overview of randomization techniques: An unbiased assessment of outcome in clinical research. J Hum Reprod Sci. 2011;4(1):8-11.

17. Mills EJ, Chan AW, Wu P, Vail A, Guyatt GH, Altman DG. Design, analysis, and presentation of crossover trials. Trials. 2009;30(10):27.

18. Aagaard A, Godiksen S, Teglers PT, Schiodt M, Glenert U. Comparison between new saliva stimulants in patients with dry mouth: a placebo-controlled double-blind crossover study. Journal of Oral Pathology and Medicine. 1992;21(8):376-80.

19. Andersson G, Johansson G, Attstrom R, Edwardsson S, Glantz PO, Larsson K. Comparison of the effect of the linseed extract Salinum and a methyl cellulose preparation on the symptoms of dry mouth. Gerodontology. 1995;12(1):12-7.

20. Bots CP, Brand HS, Veerman EC, Korevaar JC, Valentijn-Benz M, Bezemer PD et al. Chewing gum and a saliva substitute alleviate thirst and xerostomia in patients on haemodialysis. Nephrology Dialysis Transplantation. 2005;20(3):578-84.

21. Bots CP, Brand HS, Veerman EC, Valentijn-Benz M, Van Amerongen BM, Nieuw Amerongen AV et al. The management of xerostomia in patients on haemodialysis: comparison of artificial saliva and chewing gum. Palliative Medicine. 2005;19(3):202- 7.

22. Furness S, Worthington HV, Bryan G, Birchenough S, McMillan R. Interventions for themanagement of drymouth: topical therapies. Cochrane Database of Systematic Reviews 2011, Issue 12. Art. No.: CD008934.

23. Benrachou N. Etude des caracteristiques physicochimiques et de la composition biochimique d'huiles d'olive issues de trois cultivars de l'Est algerien [These]. Biochimie appliquéee: Annaba; 2013. 112p.

24. Hrobjartsson A, Gotzsche PC. Is the placebo powerless? An analysis of clinical trials comparing placebo with no treatment. N Engl J Med. 2001;344(21):1594-1602.

25. Georges D. Pathologies generales et salive [These]. Chirurgie dentaire: Nancy; 2012. 272p.

26. Lucas L, Russell A, Keast R. Molecular mechanisms of inflammation. Antiinflammatory benefits of virgin olive oil and the phenolic compound oleocanthal. Curr Pharm Des. 2011;17(8):754-68.

27. Alemany R, Navarro MA, Vogler O, Perona JS, Osada J, Ruiz-Gutierrez V. Olive oils modulate fatty acid content and signaling protein expression in apolipoprotein E knockout mice brain. Lipids. 2010;45(1):53-61.

28. Dell'Agli M, Fagnani R, Galli GV, Maschi O, Gilardi F, Bellosta S et al. Olive oil phenols modulate the expression of metalloproteinase 9 in THP-1 cells by acting on nuclear factor-kappaB signaling. J Agric Food Chem. 2010;58(4):2246-52.

29. Miles EA, Zoubouli P, Calder PC. Differential anti-inflammatory effects of phenolic compounds from extra-virgin olive oil identified in human whole blood cultures. Nutrition. 2005;21(3):389-94.

30. Zhang X, Cao J, Zhong L. Hydroxytyrosol inhibits proinflammatory cytokines, iNOS, and COX-2 expression in human monocytic cells. Naunyn Schmiedebergs Arch Pharmacol. 2009;379(6):581-6.

31. Goya L, Mateos R, Bravo L. Effect of the olive oil phenol hydroxytyrosol on human hepatoma HepG2 cells. Protection against oxidative stress induced by tertbutylhydroperoxide. Eur J Nutr. 2007;46(2):70-8.

32. Owen RW, Giacosa A, Hull WE, Haubner R, Wurtele G, Spiegelhalder B et al. Olive-oil consumption and health: the possible role of antioxidants. Lancet Oncol. 2000;1(2):107-12.

33. Salvini S, Sera F, Caruso D, Giovannelli L, Visioli F, Saieva C et al. Daily consumption of a highphenol extra-virgin olive oil reduces oxidative DNA damage in postmenopausal women. Br J Nutr. 2006;95(4):742-51.

34. Servili M, Esposto S, Fabiani R, Urbani S, Taticchi A, Mariucci F et al. Phenolic compounds in olive oil: antioxidant, health and organoleptic activities according to their chemical structure. Inflammopharmacology. 2009;17(2):76-84.

35. De La Torre R. Bioavailability of olive oil phenolic compounds in humans. Inflammopharmacology. 2008;16(5): 245-7.

36. Visioli F, Caruso D, Grande S, Bosisio R, Villa M, Galli G et al. Virgin Olive Oil Study (VOLOS): vasoprotective potential of extra virgin olive oil in mildly dyslipidemic patients. Eur J Nutr. 2005;44(2):121-7.

37. Visioli F, Claudio G. Biological properties of olive oil phytochemicals. Crit Rev Food Sci Nutr. 2002;42(3):209-21.

38. Vissers MN, Zock PL, Katan MB. Bioavailability and antioxidant effects of olive oil phenols in humans: a review. Eur J Clin Nutr. 2004;58:955-65.

39. Klestov AC, Webb J, Latt D, Schiller G, McNamara K, Young DY et al. Treatment of xerostomia: a double-blind trial in 108 patients with Sjogren's syndrome. Oral Surg Oral Med Oral Pathol. 1981;51(6):594-9.

40. Donatsky O, Johnsen T, Holmstrup P, Bertram U. Effect of Saliment on parotid salivary gland secretion and on xerostomia caused by Sjogren's syndrome. Scand J Dent Res. 1982;90(2):157-62.

41. Gravenmade EJ, Vissink A. Mucin-containing lozenges in the treatment of intraoral problems associated with Sjogren's syndrome. A double-blind crossover study in 42 patients. Oral Surg Oral Med Oral Pathol. 1993;75(4):466-71.

42. Van der Reijden WA, Van der Kwaak H, Vissink A, Veerman EC, Amerongen AV. Treatment of xerostomia with polymerbased saliva substitutes in patients with Sjogren's syndrome. Arthritis Rheuma. 1996;39(1):57-63.

43. Andersson G, Johansson G, Attstrom R, Edwardsson S, Glantz PO, Larsson K. Comparison of the effect of the inseed extract Salinum and a methyl cellulose preparation on the symptoms of dry mouth. Gerodontology. 1995;12(1):12-7.

44. Johansson G, Andersson G, Edwardsson S, Bjorn AL, Manthorpe R, Attstrom R. Effects of mouthrinses with linseed extract Salinum without/with chlorhexidine on oral conditions in patients with Sjogren's syndrome. A double-blind crossover investigation. Gerodontology. 2001;18(2):87-94.

45. Momm F, Volegova-Neher NJ, Schulte-Monting J, Guttenberger R. Different saliva substitutes for treatment of xerostomia following radiotherapy. A prospective crossover study. Strahlenther Onkol. 2005;181(4):231-6.

46. Taweechaisupapong S, Pesee M, Aromdee C, Laopaiboon M, Khunkitti W. Efficacy of pilocarpine lozenge for postradiation xerostomia in patients with head and neck cancer. Aust Dent J. 2006;51(4):333-7.

47. Kim JH, Ahn JH, Choi JH, Jung DW, Kwon JS. Effect of 0.1% pilocarpine mouthwash on xerostomia: double-blind, randomised controlled trial. J Oral Rehabil. 2014;41:226-35.

48. Ship JA, McCutcheon JA, Spivakovsky S, Kerr AR. Safety and effectiveness of topical dry mouth products containing olive oil, betaine, and xylitol in reducing xerostomia for

polypharmacy-induced dry mouth. J Oral Rehabil. 2007;34(10):724-32.

49. Vivino FB, Carsons SE, Foulks G, Daniels TE, Parke A, Brennan MT, et al. New Treatment Guidelines for Sjogren's Disease. Rheum Dis Clin North Am. 2016;42(3):531-51.

50. Vivino FB, Al-Hashimi I, Khan Z, LeVeque FG, Salisbury PL 3rd , Tran-Johnson TK et al. Pilocarpine tablets for the treatment of dry mouth and dry eye symptoms in patients with Sjogren syndrome: a randomized, placebo-controlled, fixed-dose, multicenter trial. P92-01 Study Group. Arch Intern Med. 1999;159(2):174-81.

51. Katelaris CH. Pilocarpine for dry mouth and dry eye in Sjogren's syndrome. Curr Allergy Asthma Rep. 2005;5:321.

52. Petrone D, Condemi JJ, Fife R, Gluck O, Cohen S, Dalgin P. A double-blind, randomized, placebo-controlled study of cevimeline in Sjogren's syndrome patients with xerostomia and keratoconjunctivitis sicca. Arthritis Rheum. 2002;46(3):748-54.

53. Fife RS, Chase WF, Dore RK, Wiesenhutter CW, Lockhart PB, Tindall E et al. Cevimeline for the Treatment of Xerostomia in Patients With Sjogren Syndrome A Randomized Trial. Arch Intern Med. 2002;162(11):1293-300.

54. Creuzot C, Passemard M, Viau S, Joffre C, Pouliquen P, Elena PP et al. Improvement of symptomatology in patients with ocular dryness treated orally with polyunsaturated fatty acids. J Fr Ophtalmo. 2006;29(8):868-73.

55. Cury-Boaventura MF, Gorjao R, de Lima TM, Fiamoncini J, Torres RP, Mancini-Filho J et al. Effect of olive oil-based emulsion on human lymphocyte and neutrophil death. J Parenter Enteral Nutr. 2008;32(1):81-7.

56. Mena MP, Sacanella E, Vazquez-Agell M, Morales M, Fito M, Escoda R et al. Inhibition of circulating immune cell activation: a molecular antiinflammatory effect of the Mediterranean diet. Am J Clin Nutr. 2009;89(1):248-56.

57. Puertollano MA, Puertollano E, Alvarez de Cienfuegos G, de Pablo MA. Significance of olive oil in the host immune resistance to infection. Br J Nutr. 2007;98(Suppl1):54-8.

58. Romero C. News release, American Chemical Society. J Agric Food Chem. 2007;55: 680-6.

59. Giamarellos-Bourboulis EJ, Geladopoulos T, Chrisofos M, Koutoukas P, Vassiliadis J, Alexandrou I et al. Oleuropein: a novel immunomodulator conferring prolonged survival in experimental sepsis by Pseudomonas aeruginosa. Shock. 2006;26(4):410- 6.

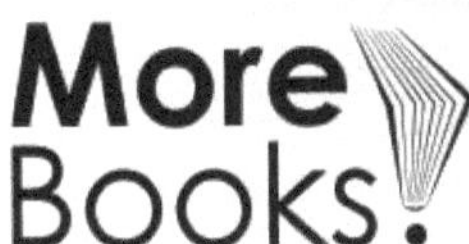

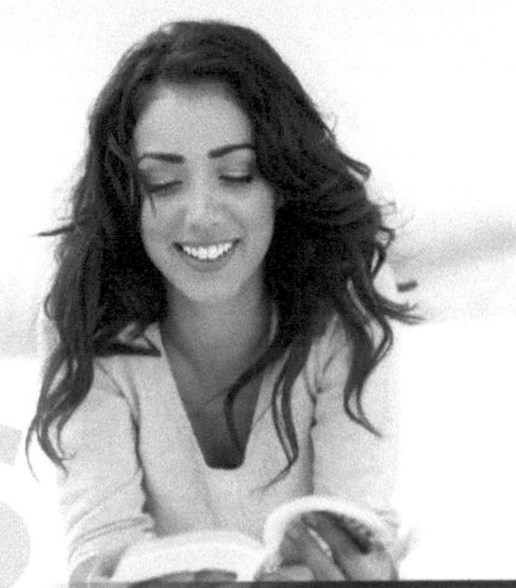

I want morebooks!

Buy your books fast and straightforward online - at one of world's fastest growing online book stores! Environmentally sound due to Print-on-Demand technologies.

Buy your books online at
www.morebooks.shop

Kaufen Sie Ihre Bücher schnell und unkompliziert online – auf einer der am schnellsten wachsenden Buchhandelsplattformen weltweit! Dank Print-On-Demand umwelt- und ressourcenschonend produziert.

Bücher schneller online kaufen
www.morebooks.shop

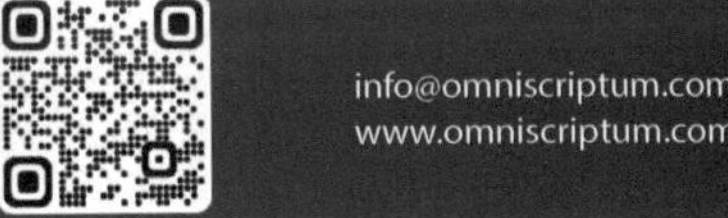

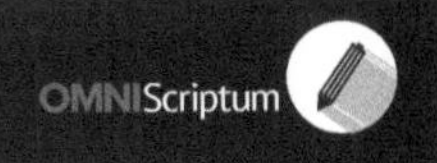

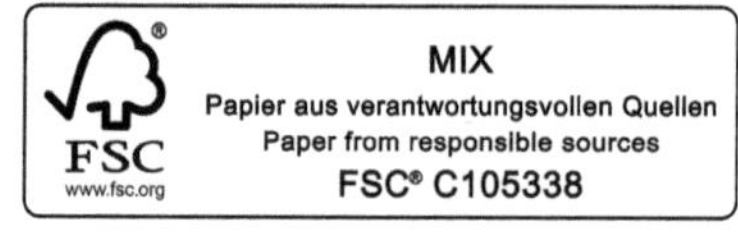

Printed by Books on Demand GmbH, Norderstedt / Germany